THE ESSENTIAL POSTPARTUM EXERCISES AND NUTRITION TOOLKIT

13 Hacks to Rebuild Pelvic Strength,
Restore Energy and Nourish Your Body
with Safe Movement and Easy Meals

KACEY QUINN

CONTENTS

INTRODUCTION

In the spring of 2022, I stood in the formula aisle of yet another grocery store and stared at empty shelves. My son was still under a year old. The national formula shortage was at its worst, with stores across the country running out entirely, and I had already been to seven other stores that morning. I called my husband from the parking lot and cried. Not quietly. The kind of crying that comes from somewhere deeper than that particular moment, the kind that carries everything that has been building for months without a proper outlet.

I had already spent weeks feeling like a failure for not being able to breastfeed the way I had planned. I had tried everything, advice from my mother, my aunts, my neighbors, a lactation specialist, every book I could find, every traditional remedy passed down through generations of women who had done this before me. Nothing worked. My body simply could not produce enough milk, and eventually I had to surrender to formula, which felt at the time like admitting defeat. And then the formula ran out. Nationally. A friend of a friend, someone I barely knew, drove two hours to bring me ten cans of Enfamil because she had heard through a mutual contact that I was struggling to find any. When she pulled up, I hugged her before she could even get out of the car properly. I could not find the words. I just held on for a moment longer than was probably normal for someone I had never properly met, because in that season, that kind of generosity from a near stranger felt like the most seen I had been in months.

Something broke open in me that season. Not permanently, and not in a way that did not eventually lead somewhere useful. But it showed me clearly how enormous the gap is between what new mothers are told and what they actually need, and how completely alone most of us are when we try to navigate it, piecing together information from wherever we can find it, doing our best with whatever is within reach.

In the days after the formula crisis settled, I was not okay. The anxiety had taken a physical toll that I had not anticipated. I stopped eating properly without even realizing it, surviving on water and crackers for nearly three days while my body quietly paid the price. My blood sugar dropped low enough to send me back to my OB, weeks past my six-week checkup, feeling like I had somehow gone backwards. I sat in the waiting room thinking about how nobody had warned me. How the emotional weight of new motherhood could land so directly in your body. How depletion could sneak up on you not just from birth, but from the weeks and months following it, from anxiety and skipped meals and the relentless pressure of keeping a tiny person alive when you are barely keeping yourself together.

That visit quietly changed everything. It did not feel dramatic in the moment. But sitting in that waiting room gave me space to ask questions I had never thought to ask before. What was my body actually missing? What had pregnancy and birth taken from me that I had never replaced? And why had nobody, not my OB, not the books I had read, not one well-meaning person in my life, ever told me that what I ate and how I moved in those early months would shape how I felt, how I recovered, and how long it would take to feel like myself again?

This book came out of that gap. When I started researching what I wished I had known in those early months, I discovered that the questions I had been carrying since birth all had answers: *Why my core felt disconnected? Why my muscles still ached weeks later? Why I felt so depleted no matter what I ate?* Every one of them had a real, evidence-based explanation. The information existed. It just had not reached me when I needed it.

My first book, *The Essential Postpartum Care Toolkit*, covers the emotional and mental side of recovery, the hormonal shifts, the identity changes, and the moments when new motherhood feels nothing like you expected. This book is its companion. Where one focuses on your mind and heart, the other focuses on your body and what it actually needs to recover. Movement healing your core and pelvic floor without making things worse. Nutrition rebuilding what pregnancy and birth depleted. Practical strategies for one hand, no complicated prep, and approximately five minutes at a time.

Part I covers seven movement hacks built around where your body is right now. No crunches, no planks, no exercises adding pressure to tissue still healing. Just the breathing technique reconnecting your deep core, the pelvic floor approach most moms never receive, the posture resets preventing the aches building through months of feeding and carrying, and a safe progression telling you exactly when and how to do more.

Part II covers six nutrition hacks that address the most overlooked drivers of postpartum depletion. Mood, brain fog, tissue repair, hydration, the gap between eating and actually nourishing, and how to think clearly about supplements when you are too exhausted to research anything properly.

This book is for every postpartum mom. The one who breastfed or the one who formula fed. The one who had a C-section or the one who pushed for many hours. The first-time mom or the one on her fourth. Wherever you are in your recovery, whatever your experience looked like, there is something here for you.

I wrote this for the version of myself sitting in that waiting room, not knowing what questions to ask. If that is where you are right now, I am glad this found you!

PART I: FUNCTIONAL MOVEMENT

7 Hacks

FOUNDATION: REWIRING CORE RECOVERY

"Your body grew, nourished, and birthed a human. That is not 'damage.' That is architecture."

—Dr. Jen Gunter

I tried doing crunches six weeks postpartum. My belly didn't flatten. Instead, a strange ridge formed down the middle of my stomach, like a little mountain range. It was alarming, and nobody had warned me.

I wish someone had explained this to me before I tried those crunches. If you've heard the term diastasis recti, you might still feel confused about what it actually means. If you haven't heard it before, don't worry. Let me break down what's really happening inside your belly. During pregnancy, your abdominal muscles stretch apart down the middle to make room for your growing baby. The connective tissue between those muscles, called the linea alba, gets thin and stretched out like an overstretched rubber band. This happens to nearly every pregnant woman by the end of the third trimester. It's normal and necessary.

But what you do in those early postpartum months matters. Jump into crunches or sit-ups too soon, and you're creating pressure that pushes outward on tissue that's already weakened. Think of it like squeezing a tube of toothpaste from the middle when it's already split open. The pressure pushes your muscles farther apart instead of bringing them back together. If you see a bulge or ridge forming down the center of your belly when you try to sit up, that's called "doming." It's your body showing you the tissue isn't ready for that movement yet.

Here's what the research tells us: your linea alba keeps remodeling and strengthening for six to twelve months after birth, not six weeks *(Mota et al., 2015)*. So instead of chasing flat abs or a six-pack, think of your core as a pressure management system. Its real job is functional, not aesthetic. It supports you when you lift your baby, walk, laugh, sneeze, and go about your day. That kind of strength comes from breathing, gentle activation, and gradual progression. Not from doing a hundred crunches.

What Your Six-Week Checkup Actually Means

Your six-week postpartum checkup is an important milestone, but it's often misunderstood. Many moms walk out of that appointment believing they've been given a green light to resume all their pre-pregnancy activities. In reality, your provider is checking for the serious stuff: signs of infection, excessive bleeding, blood pressure concerns, healing of any incisions (if you had a C-section), whether your uterus has returned to its normal size, and screening for postpartum depression or anxiety. These are all critically important things to check.

But here's what they often don't assess in detail: how wide your diastasis recti gap is, whether your pelvic floor muscles are functioning properly, or if your deep core has reconnected and is working the way it should. The American College of Obstetricians and Gynecologists *(ACOG)* recommends comprehensive postpartum care, but the reality is that many six-week visits are brief and focused on ruling out serious complications *(ACOG, 2018)*.

The truth nobody tells you? Your tissue needs way longer than six weeks to heal. That connective tissue between your abs stays in active repair mode for six months to a full year. Your pelvic floor needs similar time, whether you pushed during delivery or had a C-section.

So when your provider says you're "cleared for exercise," they mean you're stable enough to gradually start moving again. It's permission for gentle reconditioning. Not high-intensity workouts or heavy lifting. Think starting line, not finish line.

Here's something important to remember: you should feel empowered to ask your provider specific questions at your six-week visit. Don't just accept a general "you're cleared." Ask things like, "How does my diastasis recti look? Should I be concerned about the width of the gap?" or "Do you have any concerns about my pelvic floor function?" or "When would you recommend I see a pelvic floor physical therapist?" These questions help you get the information you actually need. Many providers will appreciate that you're taking an active role in your recovery. And if they don't assess these things during your visit, it's okay to request a referral to someone who specializes in postpartum rehabilitation.

Know When to Stop vs. When to Push

As you work through these hacks, pay attention to what your body is telling you. Some sensations are normal. Others are warning signs that you need to pause or modify.

Stop immediately if you notice:

- New pelvic heaviness or a bulging feeling

- Your belly forming a ridge or "cone" shape during movement

- Leaking urine or stool that wasn't happening before

- Sharp pain in your abdomen or pelvis

- Increased bleeding (bright red, not just spotting)

These aren't signs of weakness. They're your body telling you to slow down.

It's normal to feel:

- Gentle muscle fatigue after exercise

- Mild soreness the next day

- Your muscles working during movement

- A little shaky during holds

The difference? Normal sensations fade quickly with rest. Warning signs stick around or get worse. If something feels wrong, trust that instinct and listen to your body. Pause, rest, and if it continues, call your provider or find a pelvic floor physical therapist.

What These Seven Hacks Will Give You

The next seven hacks are designed to work with your healing body, not against it. No crunches. No planks. No exercises that create downward pressure on weakened tissue. Just practical, doable strategies that fit into the chaos of new motherhood.

Hack 1 – The 360° Breath: teaches you how to use your breath to activate the deepest layers of your core. This is your foundation for everything else.

Hack 2 – The Pelvic Floor Lift: shows you specific techniques for strengthening your pelvic floor without overdoing it. You'll learn the difference between helpful activation and harmful clenching.

Hack 3 – The Postpartum Posture Reset: explains why your posture matters more than you think and how to reset it throughout your day, especially during feeding and babywearing.

Hack 4 – Safe Lifting Strategies: gives you the techniques to lift your baby, car seat, stroller, and everything else without straining your back or core. You'll learn the "glute squeeze" method that changes everything.

Hack 5 — Gentle Mobility Flows: introduces movement patterns that restore mobility and strength without risk. Perfect for those early months when you're still healing but want to move your body.

Hack 6 — Restorative Practices: covers the often-overlooked recovery tools like rest, stress management, and nervous system regulation. Healing isn't just about exercise.

Hack 7 — Progressive Core Loading: gives you a clear, safe progression path for building core strength over time. You'll know exactly when and how to advance without guessing.

None of these require a gym membership, special equipment, or much time. They're designed for real life with a newborn. Short, doable, and effective. Most can be done while holding your baby, during feeding time, or in the random five-minute windows that appear throughout your day.

Your body did something extraordinary. It grew, nourished, and birthed a human being. That stretched tissue, that separated gap, those weakened muscles are not damage. They are the architecture of creation. Healing starts with reconnecting to your body, and that connection begins with breath. In Hack 1, you will learn the 360° breathing technique that activates your core without a single crunch, and why this simple practice is the foundation for everything that follows.

Hack 1: The 360° Breath

"Breath is the bridge which connects life to consciousness, which unites your body to your thoughts."

—Thích Nhất Hạnh

I had my son without any medication. No epidural, no induction, nothing. Eighteen hours of contractions and forty-five minutes of pushing, entirely on my own terms. I had done my research, I knew what I wanted, and I trusted my body to handle what it was built to do.

What I did not expect was still feeling it four weeks later.

The aching in my muscles had not gone away the way I thought it would. Picking up my son one afternoon, just lifting him from the floor to my shoulder, I felt it through my whole core, a heaviness and effort that surprised me. I had assumed that choosing a natural birth meant my body would bounce back on a natural timeline. What I had not understood yet was that the birth itself was only part of the story. The muscles that had worked for eighteen hours needed something more intentional than just time and willpower to find their way back.

That is what this hack begins to address. Before we talk about strength or fitness or any of the goals that feel far away right now, we start with something your body can do this very moment, wherever you are sitting or lying down. We start with the breath.

What 360° Breathing Actually Is:

Most of us breathe into our chest, especially when we're stressed or exhausted. Our shoulders lift, our neck tenses, and only the top portion of our lungs fills with air. This shallow breathing keeps us in a low-grade stress response and does nothing to activate the deep core muscles that need attention after pregnancy.

360° diaphragmatic breathing uses your entire torso. Your diaphragm is a large, dome-shaped muscle that sits under your lungs. When it contracts during a proper inhale, it moves downward and your ribcage expands outward in all directions: front, sides, and back. Your belly rises softly. It's called 360° breathing because the expansion happens all the way around your midsection, not just in front.

This breathing pattern activates your transverse abdominis, the deepest layer of abdominal muscle that wraps around your trunk like a corset. It also engages your pelvic floor in a coordinated way. When you inhale deeply, your diaphragm lowers and your pelvic floor gently releases and lengthens. When you exhale, both naturally rebound upward together. This coordinated movement between your diaphragm and pelvic floor is part of what's called your "inner core system" (*Sapsford et al., 2001*). After pregnancy and birth, this system often stops working automatically. You have to retrain it, and breathing is where that retraining begins.

How to practice 360° diaphragmatic breathing:

1. Find a comfortable position. Lying on your back with bent knees, feet flat (an easy position for most postpartum moms). If you had a C-section and lying flat is uncomfortable, prop yourself up with pillows. The goal is to be comfortable enough that you can relax and focus.

2. Place one hand on your lower belly, the other on your ribcage. Close your

eyes if it helps you tune in.

3. Inhale slowly through your nose, feeling your rib cage widen to the sides and back as your belly rises softly. Don't force your belly—let it expand as air fills your lungs. Imagine you're filling a barrel that expands evenly in all directions, not just a balloon inflating in front of you.

4. Exhale gently through your mouth or nose. Feel your belly flatten and your ribs move back together. Try to make your exhale slightly longer than your inhale. Repeat for five to ten slow breaths.

5. Watch for common mistakes. Are you lifting your shoulders? Arching your back? Only pushing your belly forward without expanding your ribs to the sides? Breathing too quickly? If you catch yourself doing any of these, pause, reset, and try again. No judgment, just adjustment.

Helpful tips:

- Imagine air moving toward your hip bones and the sides of your ribcage, not just straight down into your belly.

- Place your hands on the sides of your ribs to physically feel that outward expansion.

- Try placing a light scarf or resistance band around your ribcage and push it outward with your breath. This tactile feedback can make the concept click faster.

How often and when to practice:

- Aim for 2-3 times daily. Each session is just 5-10 slow breaths. That's it. Quality matters more than quantity.

- Best times: First thing in the morning while you're still in bed, during any feeding session (nursing or bottle), before you go to sleep at night, or anytime you feel stressed or overwhelmed.

- When baby is sleeping: This is a great time to lie down and practice with your hands on your belly and ribs for full awareness.

- When you feel stressed: Even just 3-5 slow breaths can reset your nervous system in the moment. Use it like a pause button for your stress.

- During daily tasks: Once you get comfortable, practice while rocking your baby, waiting in line, or even while warming a bottle.

The goal isn't perfection. It's consistency. Five mindful breaths every day will serve you better than one twenty-minute session once a week that you can never find time for.

The "Baby Hug" Technique for Gentle Core Engagement

Breathing alone is powerful, but you can add a layer of gentle core engagement to make it even more effective. This is called the "Baby Hug" technique because it mimics the instinctive way you'd draw your baby close to protect them. You're not sucking in your stomach or holding your breath. You're engaging your transverse abdominis with a light, supportive squeeze.

Here's how to do it:

1. Start in a comfortable position. Lying down, sitting, or standing—whatever feels best right now. Place one hand on your lower belly.

2. Inhale slowly using your 360° breath. Let your ribs and belly expand. At the top of your inhale, pause for just a moment.

3. As you exhale, gently draw your lower belly inward. Imagine giving your baby a soft hug from the inside, or zipping up a pair of jeans that

fit snugly but comfortably. The engagement should feel internal and subtle.

4. Keep everything else relaxed. Your shoulders don't lift. Your jaw doesn't clench. Your thighs and glutes stay loose. If you notice yourself tensing everywhere or holding your breath, that's bracing, not engaging. Stop, release, and try again with less effort.

5. Repeat for 5-10 breaths. Focus on the gentle draw-in on each exhale, then fully release on each inhale.

If you're having trouble feeling the engagement, try a few tricks. Exhale with a gentle "shhh" sound. The act of making that sound naturally activates the deep core. Or place a small rolled towel under your lower back and try to reduce the pressure on it without lifting your pelvis or arching your back. Some women find it easier to feel the connection while sitting upright rather than lying down. Your body is unique. Find the cues that work for you.

Integrating Breathwork Into Your Day

You don't need a mat or quiet space for this practice; the real value comes from integrating it into daily routines—during night feeds, diaper changes, or while babywearing. Pair the Baby Hug and 360° breathing with routine caregiving moments.

During Feeding Time

Whether you're nursing or bottle-feeding, pause before you settle in. Check your shoulders. Are they up by your ears? Take three slow 360° breaths, gently engaging on each exhale. This turns feeding time into core recovery time without adding anything extra to your day.

Before Lifting Your Baby

Before you pick your baby out of the crib, bassinet, or car seat, take a microsecond to inhale and prepare. Then exhale with a gentle baby hug as you lift. This protects your back and engages your core during one of the dozens of lifts you do every single day.

While Babywearing

While you're wearing your baby in a carrier or wrap, use your breath to ground yourself. Count in for four, out for six. Let each exhale bring a tiny bit of steadiness and support to your posture.

Micro-Practice – The Secret

You don't need to do twenty minutes of breathwork on the floor. One intentional breath before you get out of bed in the morning helps more than a long session you never find time for. If you get distracted and forget for hours, that's normal. Life with a newborn is chaotic. When you remember again, just start fresh. No guilt, no judgment. Just one more breath.

Habit Stacking

Attach your breathwork to something you already do automatically. This is the best way to try habit stacking. Every time you pick up your baby, tie in a breath check. When you stand up from the couch, use that moment to inhale and engage as you rise. These actions become triggers that remind you to breathe intentionally. Even if you only remember once or twice a day at first, that's progress. Consistency builds slowly.

When Distractions Happen (And They Will)

The reality is that distractions are constant. The dog barks. Your toddler needs a snack. Someone's at the door. You'll forget to breathe deeply for entire afternoons. When this happens, and it will, don't beat yourself up. Treat each new moment as a fresh start. If you catch yourself slouching with a clenched jaw while holding your baby, that's just your body asking for attention. Pause. Take one breath. Lower your shoulders. That's enough.

Track Your Small Wins

Maybe this week you felt less tension in your upper back after feeding sessions. Maybe standing up with your baby felt more stable than it did last week. Maybe you can now sense your core engaging when you couldn't before. These shifts might seem tiny, but they're proof that the work is happening. If you want, jot quick notes on your phone so you can look back later and see how far you've come. If that feels like too much, just mentally acknowledge one moment each night where you remembered to breathe intentionally.

Troubleshooting "Doming" and Old Habits

What Is Doming?

Doming is when a ridge or bulge forms along the center of your belly during movement. It often shows up when you try to sit up from lying down, lift something heavy, or engage your core too aggressively. If you see this happening, stop. It means your tissue isn't ready for that level of intensity or that particular movement yet.

Doming looks like a small mountain or tent shape pushing up along your midline. It's easiest to spot in a mirror or by recording a quick video of yourself. Place your hand on your belly and watch what happens when you lift your head or sit up. If you see or feel that ridge forming, back off immediately.

Common Triggers:

- Traditional sit-ups or crunches

- Holding your breath during any kind of effort

- Moving too quickly without engaging first

- Attempting planks or push-ups before your core is ready

- Standing up from lying down without rolling to your side first

- Lifting your baby without exhaling and engaging

What to Do Instead:

- Roll to your side before sitting up. Never go straight from lying flat to sitting upright.

- Slow everything down. Exhale gently as you begin any effort.

- Keep movements controlled and deliberate.

- If something consistently causes doming, stop doing it and choose a gentler alternative.

Old breathing habits can sneak back in when you might find yourself reverting to chest breathing, tensing your shoulders, or using your neck muscles instead of your diaphragm. When you notice this, don't judge yourself. Just reset. Check in with yourself randomly throughout the day: Am I breathing into my ribs? Are my shoulders relaxed? If you feel tension building in your upper body, take a few moments to lie down and practice your 360° breath with your hands on your belly and ribs. That physical feedback helps break the old pattern.

Your breath is the foundation. It's what makes everything else in this book possible. And the beautiful thing? It's always with you. No equipment. No extra time carved out of your day. Just you, reconnecting with your body. When you're connected, you're teaching your body how to heal.

Your pelvic floor went through just as much as everything else during pregnancy and birth. It held the weight, it stretched, it worked quietly in the background for nine months without you ever having to think about it. Now it needs the same intentional attention you just gave your breath. Hack 2 is where that conversation finally happens.

Hack 2: Pelvic Floor Recovery Beyond the Kegel

"The pelvic floor is the foundation of our core. When it's weak, everything above it suffers."
—Dr. Sarah Duvall, Core Exercise Solutions

When I started researching my first postpartum book, I came across the term "pelvic floor" for what felt like the first time in a meaningful way. I knew the muscles existed. What I had never been told was that they needed specific, gentle exercise to recover properly after birth, and that without that intentional attention, recovery could be slower, incomplete, or quietly complicated in ways I might not even connect back to those muscles.

My OB had not mentioned it, the discharge paperwork had not covered it, and even the well-meaning family members who filled my fridge and checked on my sleep had never once brought it up.

I remember sitting with that information and feeling two things at once. Grateful that I had finally found it, and quietly frustrated that it had taken me wanting to write a book about postpartum recovery to learn something my body had needed all along.

I will say, I thought eighteen hours of labor was a lot until I read a comment on a social post from a mom who had endured almost thirty-seven hours. I was already exhausted just reading it. If you are that mom, I genuinely admire you more than words can say. And now, please keep reading, because your pelvic floor deserves even more credit than you have probably given it.

The truth is that most moms never get a proper conversation about the pelvic floor. They are handed a pamphlet about Kegels at their six-week checkup, if they are lucky, and sent back into their lives with no real understanding of what those muscles went through, why they behave the way they do after birth, or how to actually support their recovery. This hack is the conversation most of us never had.

What Your Pelvic Floor Actually Does

Your pelvic floor is a hammock of muscles that stretches from your pubic bone in front to your tailbone in back. It supports your bladder, uterus, and rectum. It helps you control when you pee and poop. It plays a role in sexual function. It also works with your diaphragm and deep core muscles to stabilize your entire trunk.

During pregnancy, these muscles stretched to accommodate your growing baby. The weight of your uterus pressed down on them for months. If you pushed during delivery, they stretched even further. If you had a C-section, the surgery itself, the bedrest, and carrying your baby afterward still affected them. Either way, they need attention.

When your pelvic floor is weak, you might experience leaking when you cough, sneeze, laugh, or exercise. You might feel heaviness or a bulge in your vagina. You might have trouble fully emptying your bladder. Sex might feel different or uncomfortable. These aren't things you just have to live with. They're signs your pelvic floor needs retraining.

But weakness isn't the only issue. Some women have pelvic floors that are too tight. This can cause pelvic pain, difficulty peeing, constipation, or pain during sex. If you're constantly "holding" those muscles without realizing it, or if you clench when you're stressed, you might have a tension problem, not a weakness problem. That's why learning to release is just as important as learning to contract.

The Elevator Exercise: Controlled Activation and Release

This exercise uses visualization and gentle engagement to build both strength and control. It's called the Elevator Exercise because you imagine your pelvic floor as an elevator that lifts through different floors, then descends smoothly back down. There's no squeezing as hard as you can. The focus is on subtlety, control, and full release.

Here's how to do it:

1. Sit comfortably with your feet flat on the floor and shoulders relaxed. You can also lie on your back with knees bent if sitting is uncomfortable, especially if you had a C-section.

2. Inhale slowly through your nose. Let your belly soften. Feel your pelvic floor gently release and lengthen as you breathe in.

3. As you exhale, gently lift your pelvic floor. Imagine an elevator lifting from the lobby to the first floor. The movement is upward and inward, like you're gently drawing everything up inside your pelvis. Don't squeeze your thighs or buttocks. Don't hold your breath. Just a light, internal lift.

4. Hold briefly at the first floor, then release completely as you inhale. Let the elevator glide back down to the lobby. Focus on that full release. Your pelvic floor should feel soft and relaxed, like you're letting go of tension.

5. Repeat for 5-10 slow lifts. Start with just two floors—up to floor one, then back down. Once that feels natural, you can progress to three or

four floors, pausing briefly at each level.

If you're having trouble sensing the movement, try these visualizations: imagine gently picking up a blueberry at your vaginal opening with an inward lift, or picture closing and lifting the openings of your vagina and anus without clenching your buttocks. Some women find it helpful to think of a drawstring gently pulling upward and inward, not outward or downward.

Advanced progression:

Once you're comfortable with two floors, try moving through multiple levels. Lift to floor one, pause. Lift to floor two, pause. Lift to floor three, pause. Then descend stepwise: floor two, pause; floor one, pause; lobby, full release. This builds fine motor control and teaches your muscles to work at different levels of intensity.

If you become shaky, lose track of your breath, or feel strain, return to two floors. This should never feel forceful. Quality matters more than how many floors you can reach.

Most new moms master the technique in theory, then lose it completely in the chaos of real life. Hack 3 is about bridging that gap, adapting pelvic floor work to fit C-section recovery, sneaking it into the moments you already have, and knowing when your body is telling you to slow down.

HACK 3: BUILDING YOUR PELVIC FLOOR FOUNDATION

"You need to work on both strength and muscle coordination for the entire system simultaneously. If you haven't restored coordination, you're only strengthening an uncoordinated system."
—Julie Wiebe, PT, DPT, Pelvic Health Physical Therapist

By the time you finish Hack 2, you have a sense of what your pelvic floor is and why it needs attention. But knowing and doing are two different things. Most moms try a few Kegels, lose track of whether they are doing them correctly, and quietly give up. This hack is about building the actual foundation, exercises that work for every recovery stage, adaptations for C-section moms, and a way of weaving pelvic floor care into the moments that already exist in your day.

The "Elevator Exercise": Gentle Activation for All Recovery Stages

Your pelvic floor went through nine months of increasing pressure, whether you pushed during delivery or had a C-section. Those muscles stretched, weakened, and changed. The standard advice – just do your Kegels – oversimplifies everything. Doing Kegels wrong can actually make things worse. Squeezing too hard, holding your breath, or never fully releasing can create tension, pain, and more leakage, not less. Instead, try the Elevator Exercise, which trains both muscle strength and the equally important skill of relaxation.

The Elevator Exercise uses visualization and gentle muscle engagement. Imagine your pelvis as the ground floor, and your pelvic floor as an elevator that gently lifts through a few floors when contracting, then descends smoothly as you release. There's no need to squeeze hard or hold your breath. Instead of a simple squeeze-and-release, you'll explore different levels of effort to build fine control.

Begin by sitting comfortably with your feet on the floor and shoulders relaxed. Inhale slowly through your nose, allowing your belly to soften. As you exhale, picture the elevator lifting from the lobby to the first floor with a gentle upward movement inside your pelvis. Hold briefly, then inhale and imagine the elevator gliding back down, fully releasing tension. Start with just two floors – up and down – until it feels natural.

Once comfortable, expand to three or four floors. On your exhale, gently lift your pelvic floor to floor two or three, pausing briefly at each level to sense that lift. Avoid gripping your thighs or buttocks – if you catch those muscles working, reset and use less effort. The intention is always **up and in**, not out or down. On each inhale, focus on letting go completely. **Controlled relaxation** is just as important as the lift, since holding tension all day can lead to issues like pain, trouble emptying the bladder, or more leakage *(van Reijn-Baggen et al., 2022)*.

If you're ready for a challenge, add another floor. Move gradually: lift to floor one, pause; then to floor two, pause; then descend, stepwise. This advanced progression should always be gentle and never involve breath-holding or strain. If you become shaky or lose track of your breath, return to two levels.

Technique matters. Sensory imagery can help: imagine gently picking up a blueberry at your vaginal opening with an inward lift, avoiding squeezing your thighs or buttocks. If you feel your breath catch or notice you're pushing outward, pause and reset. The movement should be a smooth, inward glide – never a forceful clamp or a push down.

Common mistakes include tensing the glutes or inner thighs, **holding your breath** (which increases pressure), or bearing down like straining on the toilet. If you notice any of these, relax and restart with gentler effort. Quality matters far more than quantity – focus on the connection and the sensation of real support.

Reflection Prompt: Elevator Check-In

After practicing, jot a quick note about how the lift and release felt. Noticing these details will help you spot recovery patterns and interrupt unhelpful habits early.

- Where did you sense effort – pelvic floor, thighs, or buttocks?

- Was releasing harder than lifting?

- What felt different compared to last time?

This exercise works anywhere – while rocking your baby, sitting in traffic, or brushing your teeth. Learning to both activate and relax your pelvic floor builds not only strength, but lasting comfort and control for the years ahead *(van Reijn-Baggen et al., 2022)*.

C-Section Variations: How to Adapt When Sitting or Standing Is Hard

Having a C-section doesn't mean skipping pelvic floor care. Carrying your baby, the surgery, and bedrest all affect the pelvic floor – sometimes in surprising ways. Scar sensitivity, numbness, or unexpected twinges can make everyday positions like sitting uncomfortable or even painful. In those early postpartum days, simply getting out of bed or laughing might tug on your incision. Maybe you're there now, inching into a position that doesn't hurt, bracing for any movement that feels stitched together tight.

If sitting hurts or your incision is tender, standard exercises may feel inaccessible. Instead, shift to **side-lying or semi-reclined positions**. Lying on your side with a pillow between your knees relieves pressure on your abdomen and lets your pelvis relax. Here, you can practice gentle pelvic floor engagement with less tension on the scar. You don't need to sit up tall or brace your core – just let your torso rest and explore subtle movement deep in the pelvis.

If side-lying isn't an option, try a semi-reclined spot in bed or on the couch. Use pillows to support your back at a comfortable angle. If your abdomen feels tight, sliding a towel under your knees can help. A warm (not hot) pack on the lower belly can relax everything enough for a few gentle contractions.

Standing may feel tough in the first weeks. If you can only manage privacy while standing, use a sink or wall for support. Lean lightly, soften your knees, and stand with feet wide for stability. Don't lock your legs or squeeze your glutes – just breathe and gently sense the pelvic floor moving. There's no rush and no pressure to hold longer than feels comfortable.

Supporting your scar is key when practicing movement. If you feel pulling or burning, fold a towel and press it gently against your lower belly, especially when standing or changing positions. **High-waisted leggings** or postpartum wraps can add gentle compression, but remove them if there's pinching or irritation. Comfort matters most – not restriction.

Pain and altered sensation are part of recovery. You may have numb spots, pins-and-needles, or areas where nothing seems to happen during pelvic floor exercises. Nerves take time to recover after surgery. Some muscles respond more quickly than others, and early progress may be uneven. Sometimes you can contract but not release, or vice versa.

Recovery is not a straight line. Some days feel easier, others more challenging. The most important thing is to stay patient and curious rather than frustrated. If pain or fatigue flare up, skip the exercise and try again later. Even imagining the pelvic floor moving can help reconnect mind and muscle.

Needing props or added support for longer than someone else is completely normal – every C-section recovery is different. When cleared by your provider, gentle **scar massage** can also help restore mobility and make pelvic floor work easier over time *(Stone, 2021)*.

Adapting exercises for your comfort is not only allowed, it's encouraged *(Stone, 2021)*. The real goal isn't perfection – it's a gradual return to bodily confidence, regaining awareness, mobility, and comfort with how your body moves as you recover.

Everyday Pelvic Floor Stacking: Integrating Rehab Into Lifting, Sneezing, and Stairs

You probably don't have time to lie on the floor and count out slow contractions while your little one cries nearby. What made the biggest difference wasn't a perfect routine or even remembering to exercise at all. It was weaving pelvic floor support into the fabric of a regular day. This is what I call **stacking**: using every-day moments to practice quick, intentional contractions, turning the things you already do into opportunities for pelvic floor rehab. Lifting your baby, sneezing, climbing stairs. You don't need privacy, a yoga mat, or even a full minute.

Start with the high-risk moves that trip up most new moms: lifting anything heavy (babies, strollers, car seats), sneezing, coughing, laughing, and climbing stairs. These are the moments when leaks or feelings of heaviness like to sneak up. Before you pick up your baby, pause for just a microsecond. Breathe in naturally, then as you exhale, gently draw your pelvic floor upward and inward. Imagine zipping up a snug pair of jeans from the inside out, subtle but supportive. Keep your jaw and shoulders loose. As you lift, maintain that gentle engagement until the effort is done, then let go completely.

When climbing stairs or standing from a chair, use the same cue: exhale, activate, move. Sneezing and coughing always seem to strike when you're least prepared. If you feel a sneeze coming on, brace just before it hits by tightening softly upward –

not clenching all-out. If it catches you off guard, don't panic. These missed moments are not failures; they're reminders for next time. Laughing, especially those sudden bursts, can challenge even the strongest pelvic floors. If you remember in time, give a quick lift as you laugh; if not, just smile and try again.

The magic of stacking is that you're building dozens of mini-reps into your day without carving out extra time. Think of every diaper pick-up, stroller hoist, or stair climb as a practice opportunity, not a chore, but an act of self-care scattered through your real life. Over time, these repetitions build muscle memory, and your body starts to support itself automatically during effort.

Sometimes you'll forget altogether, maybe you're half-awake or distracted. That's normal. There's no penalty for missing a contraction or two (or ten). Just reset when you remember. The next time you lift your baby or stand from the couch, pause for an instant and try again. Consistency counts more than perfection.

Here's what's worth knowing sooner rather than later: there's such a thing as overdoing it with pelvic floor work. You don't need to clench all day or hold contractions every moment. This can lead to tension, pain, and even more weakness over time. Brief, purposeful lifts with full release work best. Think "on" for effort, "off" the rest of the time.

If you wonder whether you're doing too much or too little, use this rule of thumb: activate for effort when lifting, pushing, or standing, and let go when it's over. Never hold tension for more than a few seconds unless specifically advised by a specialist. If your muscles feel tired or sore by evening, that's your cue to back off tomorrow.

Visual cues help. Place a sticky note on the fridge or car seat handle with a simple word, "lift" or "zip," to trigger action without thought. Some moms set phone reminders until it becomes automatic. Others tie stacking to routines: every diaper change equals one pelvic floor check-in.

If lifting brings on leaks despite your best efforts, try engaging more gently or starting the contraction slightly earlier in the move. If you notice hip tension or back strain, it could mean you're recruiting other muscles instead of the pelvic floor. Pause and reset with less effort next time. Over time, these small actions create real change. Fewer surprises with sneezing, more confidence picking up your baby, and a sense that things are finally working together again.

Signs of Overdoing: When to Pause or Seek Pelvic PT Help

Recovery in the fourth trimester is rarely consistent. One day you might feel capable; the next, unexpectedly off. It's worth knowing the difference between typical muscle fatigue and symptoms that signal something needs attention. Many new moms are left to guess, questioning whether soreness means progress or something to watch. The key is learning to trust your body's signals, especially when tiredness makes everything blur together.

Pay attention to signs your pelvic floor is being pushed too far. Increased pelvic heaviness, a weight or dropping sensation low in your pelvis, is a reason to pause. Notice new or worsening **leakage** (urine or stool), as this suggests your muscles need a break. Any **sharp pain** in your pelvis, groin, or lower back during or after movement shouldn't be dismissed as just part of recovery. Bulging or a ballooning feeling in your vagina might signal **prolapse**, which needs attention. None of these mean something is permanently wrong. They are simply your body's way of saying it needs more time and gentler movement.

Muscle tiredness is expected, especially as you rebuild after pregnancy. Mild fatigue that makes your pelvic floor feel worked but not painful should resolve in a few hours or after a night's sleep. What isn't normal: symptoms that worsen with each session, don't improve with rest, or are accompanied by ongoing discomfort, increased bleeding, throbbing, or a deep ache that lingers. Pushing harder won't speed recovery.

If symptoms flare or you hit a wall, stop exercising immediately. Lie down for true rest, no multitasking. The next day, try a gentler variation of the exercise that triggered the problem. For example, do pelvic floor activations while lying on your side instead of standing. If symptoms resolve after rest and easier movements, progress slowly and monitor how your body feels. If issues persist or worsen even after backing off, seek help.

Reaching out to a pelvic floor physical therapist is not defeat. It's a proactive step toward recovery. PTs are trained to distinguish between normal recovery and issues that need extra support. They can review your unique situation and teach adaptations beyond what any book can cover. Many moms need just one or two sessions to course-correct. There's no shame in asking for guidance; most PTs wish moms wouldn't wait until symptoms are severe.

Finding the right PT is straightforward. Your OB or midwife can often recommend trusted physios. National physiotherapy associations have searchable directories, and a quick search for "pelvic floor PT near me" is a good starting point. Telehealth has also made support more accessible, especially if in-person visits are challenging with a newborn.

Keeping a symptom log can help. Note what you feel and when, especially if symptoms shift with activity or time of day. This makes communicating with your provider much easier and helps identify patterns that might otherwise be hard to describe.

Most new mothers need support at some point. Asking for help is self-care, not a shortcoming. Strength shows up in pausing, adjusting, and seeking expert input when needed.

Red Flags: When to Pause and Get Support

- New heaviness or bulging in the pelvic region

- New leakage (urine or fecal) during activity

- Sharp pelvic pain with or after movement

- Increased bleeding after exercise

- Deep persistent ache that doesn't resolve with rest

If any of these occur, treat yourself kindly and seek advice promptly.

Most new moms are told to "just do their exercises" without ever being shown how to check if those exercises are actually working. Hack 4 changes that. We'll walk through the two-finger test together so you know exactly where your core is starting from before you push any further.

HACK 4: HOW TO MEASURE YOUR DIASTASIS

---

*"Our abdominal muscles are rarely 'broken'; rather, their weakness
is a reflection of how little we use our entire body."*
—Katy Bowman, M.S., Diastasis Recti

The Two-Finger Test

It's a strange feeling, reaching down to check the space in your own belly. Most of us never thought we'd be measuring our abs at home, yet here we are, trying to get answers that our rushed six-week checkup skipped right over. Understanding where you're starting – the width and depth of your core separation – is the first step in taking back control of your recovery. There's no shame in the numbers. This is simply your body showing you where it needs support.

Let's walk through it together. Find a quiet moment, maybe while your baby naps or plays nearby. Then follow these steps:

1. Lie flat on your back with your knees bent and feet resting on the floor. Place a small pillow or folded towel under your head to keep your neck comfortable.

2. Support your head lightly with one hand as you lift, keeping your neck relaxed.

3. Still lying on your back, place your fingertips (index and middle finger) about one finger-width above your belly button. Point them toward your toes, not side to side, so they run along the midline of your abdomen.

4. Take a slow breath in. As you exhale, gently lift just your head and shoulders off the floor, the tiniest crunch, only enough to engage the muscles, not strain them.

5. Gently press your fingertips downward into your belly. You're feeling for a soft gap or groove running down the center. Press just enough to sense whether there's space between your muscles. Don't push hard.

6. Count how many fingers fit side by side into that gap. One finger? Two? Three or more? That number is your starting measurement. Also notice how the tissue feels under your fingers. Is it firm and springy, or soft and squishy like jelly? Both the width and the feel matter.

For most new moms, a gap of up to two finger-widths is considered within normal range after pregnancy. A gap wider than two fingers, three or even four, is a sign of diastasis recti *(Sperstad et al., 2016)*. But don't stop at width. Pay attention to what's under your fingers: is the tissue firm and springy, or soft and squishy? Firm tension means the **linea alba** is recovering well. Squishiness or a deep sink-in feeling means it's still stretched and needs time and gentle support.

Now move your hand and repeat the test one to two inches above the belly button, then below it. Each spot may feel different. Some moms find the widest gap above the navel, others right at or below it. Checking all three locations gives you a complete picture of where your core needs the most attention.

Measuring both **width** (how many fingers fit) and **depth** (how far you can press down) matters. A wide but shallow gap with good tension often progresses faster than a narrow but deep, squishy separation. Recovery is not just about closing the space. It's about regaining firmness across that tissue so your core can support you in daily life *(Lee and Hodges, 2016)*. This is why some women with a small gap still struggle with back pain or weakness. It's not just the numbers; it's the quality of the tissue.

For tracking, grab a notebook or use your phone. Jot down width and tissue feel at each of the three spots, above, at, and below the navel. Check every one to two weeks. Even small shifts can feel invisible in the moment but become meaningful when you look back over several weeks.

If you feel frustrated after checking, know that a gap is common, more common than not, especially in the first months postpartum *(Sperstad et al., 2016)*. Your core went through tremendous stretching to grow a baby. With gentle attention and safe movement, these numbers can and often do improve.

Reflection Prompt: Your Core Check-In

Take a moment after measuring to write down what surprised you—good or bad:

- Did you expect more tension?

- Was the gap smaller than you feared?

- How did it feel emotionally to check?

These notes can help you track not just physical changes but how your mindset shifts with each step forward.

Seated and Lying Movements: No-Equipment Routines for Early Recovery

Early postpartum, even standing can feel exhausting, let alone "working out." But rebuilding your core doesn't require equipment or elaborate moves. Gentle exercises from your bed or living room floor are enough to begin real recovery.

Seated Marching

1. Sit tall in a sturdy chair or on your bed, feet hip-width apart, shoulders stacked over hips.

2. Take a slow **360° breath** – ribs expanding in all directions.

3. As you exhale, softly draw your belly toward your spine. Shoulders stay down, face relaxed.

4. Slowly lift one knee a few inches, pause, then lower. Switch legs, moving in a slow, steady rhythm.

C-section note: _Avoid leaning back. Place a pillow behind your lower back if needed, and stop if you feel any pulling near your scar._

Lying Heel Slides

1. Lie on your back, knees bent, feet flat on the floor, arms at your sides.

2. Inhale to expand your ribs, then exhale and softly draw your belly in.

3. Slowly slide one heel along the floor, straightening your leg while keeping your lower back pressed down.

4. Inhale as you return your heel to the start position.

5. Alternate legs for **8–10 reps** each side. If you see **doming** (a ridge along your midline) or feel pelvic pressure, stop and reset.

C-section note: _This movement is usually comfortable by weeks two or three. Don't push through discomfort. If unsure, simply bend and straighten the knee without the slide._

Supine Pelvic Tilts

1. Lie on your back, knees bent, feet hip-width apart. Place your hands on your hips or belly.

2. Breathe in, then exhale as you gently tilt your pelvis, pressing your lower back into the floor. Your tailbone tips slightly upward.

3. Hold for one to two seconds, then release back to neutral.

4. Repeat 10–12 times, moving slowly and mindfully. This move helps reconnect you with deep abdominal muscles and eases lower-back tension.

C-section note: *Place a small folded towel under your hips if you feel wobbly or uncomfortable.*

It's normal to hold your breath, let your stomach dome, or move too quickly at first. If any of these happen, pause, take a slow 360° breath, and start again. If something causes pain, back off completely.

These movements fit naturally into your day – seated marching while your baby is in a bouncer, heel slides during tummy time, pelvic tilts before bed or after feedings. Two or three minutes scattered throughout the day adds up more than you'd expect.

Early postpartum exercise is about consistency and connection, not intensity. Focus less on perfect reps and more on gentle body awareness. Rest when tired. Even two heel slides is progress.

Progression Paths: When and How to Advance Safely

At some point, heel slides and seated marches will start to feel easy. That's a good sign – and it raises a fair question: how do you know when you're ready for more?

The answer isn't about how many weeks have passed. It's about what your body is telling you. You're **ready to advance** when you can hold gentle core engagement through each rep without belly bulging, **doming**, or shaking. When basic movements no longer cause **leaking**, instability, or back pain. When you can exhale and engage during movement, not hold your breath through it. These markers matter far more than any external timeline.

When you see them, add new challenges gradually. Start small: hold a lightweight object – a folded towel or empty laundry basket – during seated marching and see if your core stays steady. If it does, add reps or try a slightly harder variation the following week. Move from lying to seated to standing only when each level feels solid. Mini-squats and gentle standing marches are good next steps. Keep a hand on your belly for feedback – if you feel doming or your core giving way, step back to easier movements until control returns.

Advancing too fast, especially with diastasis recti, can cause setbacks. If doming returns in new movements, or you notice heaviness, pressure, or leaking, slow down. Return to simpler exercises until symptoms resolve. Setbacks after rough nights, growth spurts, extra lifting, or illness are normal – they don't erase your progress. They just mean your body needs a reset before moving forward.

A good rule of thumb: if you can perform a movement well for **three consecutive days** with no symptoms, you're likely ready for the next challenge. If new pain appears – incision discomfort, sharp pelvic pain, or unusual fatigue – back off and protect what you've built.

Your real-world milestones matter most: lifting your baby without bracing, rolling out of bed with control, laughing without leaking. Every one of those is genuine progress worth tracking.

Progress Tracker: Weekly Checklist

- Can I do all basic moves (heel slides, pelvic tilts, seated marches) without bulging or pain?

- Have I added light resistance (like a laundry basket) without losing core control?

- Did any new symptoms appear (leaking, heaviness, back pain)?

- Did I feel steady and strong for three consecutive days?

- If I had setbacks, did I scale back and recover?

Check off each "yes" as you go—progress often happens with small, steady wins.

Core Check-Ins: Tracking Milestones and Celebrating Small Wins

Making sense of your progress with diastasis recti can feel overwhelming, especially when every day seems different. You might wonder if you're actually getting anywhere or just going in circles.

One thing that helps is setting up a simple, consistent routine for core check-ins. Checking in weekly or every other week is enough – too often, and tiny shifts get lost; too far apart, and it's easy to forget what's actually improved. Pick a day that works for you, maybe Sunday night after the baby's asleep or Monday morning before breakfast. Keep it consistent, but don't stress if you miss a week.

For each check-in, note the width and tissue feel of your gap at the three spots you measured earlier – above, at, and below the navel. Also note how well you can engage your deep core on the exhale. Is it easier than last time? You might rate tissue tension as **squishy**, **firming**, or **springy** to track change over time. Numbers matter, but so does how things feel under your fingertips.

Physical milestones are important, but the biggest wins often show up quietly in daily life. Less back pain when lifting your baby from the crib. Rolling out of bed without that awkward struggle. Rising from the floor with more control. Write these down, even if they seem small – "lifted the car seat without bracing" or "sneezed without leaking" are real markers of progress. Over time, these notes remind you how far you've come, even when the gap itself is slow to change.

Don't underestimate emotional validation during this process. Every week or two, give yourself credit for what you've done – write down three things you're proud of that have nothing to do with numbers. Maybe it's sticking with your check-ins, remembering to breathe during a tough moment, or simply being patient with slow progress. Sometimes I wrote, "I showed up for myself this week," and that was enough. Your effort counts whether or not you hit a specific milestone.

There will be weeks when progress stalls or slips backward – after sleepless nights, extra carrying, or a particularly hard stretch. Recovery isn't a straight line. If you hit a plateau or notice new symptoms like doming, heaviness, or pain, pause and assess. Did anything change in your routine? Did you push harder than usual? If so, return to basics for a week or two. Regaining stability now prevents bigger setbacks later.

If plateaus last several weeks or symptoms worsen, reaching out to a pelvic floor physical therapist is a wise next step. A professional can spot something you might have missed or suggest small adjustments that make a real difference. Slowing down or pausing certain exercises during tough stretches doesn't set you back – often, you return stronger and more aware.

Nobody else's timeline matters here. Social media skips the quiet work and jumps straight to the after. Your recovery is happening in real life – in kitchen chairs, on living room floors, between diaper changes and late-night feeds. That's worth something.

Measuring your core tells you where you're starting from. But what about everything happening above it? Hours of feeding, holding, and hunching take a toll that no finger test can catch. Hack 5 tackles the nursing slouch and the simple resets that keep your upper body from paying the price.

HACK 5: THE NURSING SLOUCH FIX

"Exercise won't change the way you move. You have to change the way you move, and that can improve how muscles function."
—Dr. Shirley Sahrmann, PT, PhD, Washington University School of Medicine

There is a specific kind of exhaustion that lives in your upper back. Not the tired arms from carrying your baby, not the foggy head from broken sleep, but the deep, grinding ache between your shoulder blades that builds quietly over weeks of hunching forward during every feed. I felt it whether I was bottle feeding, burping, or just sitting with my son in my arms trying to keep him settled. It took me longer than I would like to admit to connect those afternoon headaches and that locked feeling in my neck to how I was sitting during every single feed. Posture felt like a yoga class concern, not a recovery one. This hack is the one I wish someone had handed me in the very first week.

The "Shoulder Stack": Rebuilding Upper Body Support While Feeding

There's a moment, often in the early hours, when you feel how heavy your body is. Shoulders rounded, neck aching, upper back burning as you cradle your baby yet again. Most new moms unknowingly spend hours twisted into awkward positions to keep their baby comfortable. This "nursing slouch" is more than a bad habit. Over time, frequent poor posture leaves you stiff, sore, and disconnected from your own comfort. I remember hunching in the same chair, my back aching with every feed, my focus always on my baby rather than myself. A few simple adjustments changed everything.

The **Shoulder Stack** is a quick reset for marathon feeding sessions. It requires no special gear, just mindful setup before each feed:

1. Place your feet flat on the floor, knees bent about ninety degrees.

2. Sit all the way back so your hips are fully supported by the chair.

3. Relax your shoulders, letting them drop naturally. Roll them up toward your ears, then glide them gently back and down.

4. Imagine stacking your shoulder blades directly over your hips, building a stable pillar through your core.

5. Open your chest naturally and tuck your chin slightly so your ears align over your shoulders.

6. If your head juts forward, gently draw it back until you feel tall but not stiff.

To make this setup sustainable, use whatever pillows or towels you have available. Use a nursing pillow or any firm pillow to bring the baby up to your breast or bottle, not the other way around. Tuck a thin pillow or rolled towel behind your lower back for extra lumbar support. This small change is especially helpful if you're recovering from a C-section or dealing with core soreness. If your chair feels too deep or soft, place another pillow behind your upper back to help you stay upright. If needed, put a folded blanket under your feet so your knees sit at the right height. Comfort can be improvised; it doesn't need to be expensive or fancy *(Afshariani et al., 2019; Dowling et al., 2023)*.

If you slip into old habits, slumping, leaning, or letting one shoulder rise, just notice it without judging yourself. When you catch yourself off-balance, reset: plant both feet, sit tall, and even out your shoulders. If one side feels tighter, take a slow breath and relax it before recalibrating your shoulder stack. If your chin drops toward your chest, bring it back up so your gaze is forward and your neck feels spacious.

It's easy to forget about posture when you're tired or stuck in round-the-clock feeding cycles. Place sticky notes on your chair with a simple reminder: "Shoulder Stack!" or "Sit tall." A ribbon on your water bottle works too. Over time, these cues help posture checks become automatic rather than another thing to remember.

Reflection Exercise: Your Posture Reset Checklist

Before each feed, run through this quick routine:

1. Set both feet flat on the floor.

2. Sit all the way back in your chair.

3. Roll shoulders up, back, and down.

4. Stack shoulder blades over hips.

5. Place baby on pillows so you don't hunch.

6. Add a pillow behind your low back if needed.

7. Gently tuck your chin so ears align with shoulders.

Notice how you feel compared to your usual setup. Does your upper back hurt less? Is it easier to breathe? Jot down small changes in comfort after each session. Over time, these resets add up.

Micro-Stretches You Can Do with a Baby on Your Lap

Finding relief from aches can feel impossible when you're anchored with a baby on your lap, arms full and stuck in one spot. Most moms experience mounting tension in their spine, neck, and shoulders while feeding, soothing, or simply being their baby's jungle gym. But you don't need long breaks or both hands free to ease discomfort. Micro-stretches, tiny intentional movements, fit easily into the hectic rhythm of caring for a little one. Weaving these into my day made a bigger difference than I expected.

Chest Opener

1. While sitting with your baby, clasp your hands behind your back or hold opposite wrists.

2. Gently open your chest, feeling your collarbones widen and shoulder blades draw together.

3. Take three slow breaths. If clasping isn't possible, simply roll your shoulders back and down as you inhale.

Side Neck Stretch

1. Sit tall and tip your left ear toward your left shoulder.

2. Keep your shoulders relaxed and your right shoulder gently pressing down. You should feel a lengthening along the right side of your neck.

3. Hold for three to five breaths, then switch sides.

Overhead Side Reach

1. While your baby feeds or dozes, support them with one arm.

2. Reach your free arm overhead and gently lean away from it.

3. Hold for two to three breaths, feeling the stretch along your side ribs. Switch sides when you switch your baby.

Seated Torso Twist

1. While burping your baby or singing a lullaby, sit tall with both feet flat on the floor.

2. Gently swivel your torso left, then right, keeping your hips still.

3. Move slowly and only as far as feels comfortable. This releases tension around the waist and mid-back.

Seated Cat-Cow

1. Sit tall with both feet flat on the floor and your hands resting on your thighs.

2. Inhale as you arch your back gently and lift your chest, letting your shoulders roll back.

3. Exhale as you round slightly, tucking your chin if comfortable. Repeat three to five times, keeping movements gentle and within a pain-free range.

If you're recovering from a C-section or struggling with sore breasts, adjust as needed. If your incision feels tender or your lower belly is tight, avoid deep forward bends or twists. Focus instead on neck rolls or gentle shoulder shrugs. Use a soft pillow or rolled towel across your lap to protect your incision while you hold your baby and stretch. For breast discomfort, choose the Side Neck Stretch or Overhead Reach, which leave your chest uncompressed.

Use caregiving breaks as built-in reminders for movement. While waiting for a burp or rocking in a chair, scan for tension: burning between the shoulder blades after a feed, aching low back from sitting too long. Target where you feel discomfort. Gentle torso twists for the waist, soft shoulder rolls for the upper back, or subtle pelvic tilts for lower back relief. To do a pelvic tilt, simply rock your hips forward and back while seated, which soothes the back without disrupting your baby.

Pay attention to your own trouble spots. Sore wrists from cradling? Slowly circle or flex them when possible. Numbness from sitting? Shift side to side or alternately lift each foot to boost circulation. This is about tuning in, not pushing through pain.

Some days you'll manage only a couple of seconds before your baby needs you; other days, you might string together several stretches during a sleepy feed. These brief resets add up, helping you reclaim comfort without ever leaving your chair. With practice, you'll spot and ease tension earlier, before discomfort grows.

Unwinding Tech Neck:

Looking down at your phone during feeds and cuddles is completely normal. It's a lifeline for messages, support groups, and much-needed distraction during long nursing sessions. But constantly peering downward forces your head forward and piles stress onto your cervical spine. Research shows that for every inch your head moves forward, it adds roughly 10 extra pounds of force on your neck. At a 60-degree tilt, the kind most people use when scrolling, the pressure can reach up to 60 pounds *(Hansraj, 2014)*. Over repeated days and nights of feeding, that strain adds up fast.

Adjusting Your Set-Up

The most effective fix is changing your angle. Instead of curving down to meet your device, bring it up to you. Prop your phone on a pillow on your lap or use a clamp-style holder attached to your chair or couch. This keeps your chin parallel to the floor and eases strain on your neck and back. Using a tablet or e-reader? Stack it on books or a soft toy pile to raise it. During pumping, elevate your device to avoid craning. The less you bend forward, the better your muscles will feel.

Two quick movements can release tension even with a baby in your arms. No equipment needed, just one free hand and a few seconds between feeds.

Chin Tucks

1. Sit or stand with your shoulders relaxed and eyes looking forward.

2. Pull your chin straight back, creating a gentle double chin. Don't tilt your head down.

3. Hold for five breaths, then release. Repeat often throughout the day, especially after looking down at your phone or baby.

Shoulder Blade Squeezes

1. Sit tall with your arms relaxed at your sides or resting on your lap.

2. Imagine holding a pencil between your shoulder blades. Draw them gently together and down.

3. Hold for three counts, then release completely. Do these while waiting for baby to latch, during TV commercials, or as you listen to a podcast.

Tech-Free Breaks

Building pockets of tech-free time helps your body reset. Start small by unplugging during one session daily. Maybe it's the first morning feed, spent focused on your baby's breath, or an afternoon bottle with gentle breathing instead of notifications. If going completely tech-free feels like too much, set soft limits. Keep devices an arm's length away so you must lift them to eye level, use Do Not Disturb for short intervals, or swap a scroll for a book or quiet music once a day.

Making It a Habit

Try linking posture checks to daily routines. Each time you pick up your phone or finish a feed, do a chin tuck or squeeze your shoulder blades. These small habits become automatic over time, blending into your day without feeling like extra effort. Keeping tech at eye level when feeding or rocking your baby makes a real difference, as does brief but frequent movement throughout the day.

Progress Over Perfection

The goal isn't perfect posture or quitting your phone entirely. It's making small adjustments to prevent pain. In a season where so much feels uncontrollable, movement breaks and short tech pauses are a simple way to reclaim a bit of comfort without sacrificing connection or sanity.

Posture Checkpoints: Building Awareness with Mirrors and Selfies

Noticing your posture in the middle of exhausted motherhood is genuinely hard. Most of the time, you're unaware of how you're sitting until the ache becomes constant. One surprisingly effective habit is using tools you already have. A mirror and your phone can show you how you're actually sitting, holding, or feeding. Don't pose. Just snap a quick side or front photo of your natural position during a feed. Do your shoulders curve forward? Is your head jutting out? Is your back rounding more than you realized? This visual feedback makes it much easier to spot the habits that lead to later discomfort.

Mirrors are just as effective. Keep a small mirror nearby, or use a hallway one, for quick alignment checks after feeds or before standing up. Even a fast glance can tell you if you're leaning, twisting, or letting your shoulders hike up. Picking a regular time, like after breakfast or before a nap, to check your reflection for just ten seconds can help without any self-criticism involved.

Let technology work for you. Set recurring phone alarms labeled "Posture Check" at key times during the day. These reminders interrupt autopilot and cue you to quickly scan your body for tension or imbalance. Some moms prefer habit-tracking apps that send random nudges; others like sticky notes on the fridge or bathroom mirror. The point is to make reminders noticeable, especially on tough, tiring days.

A mental head-to-toe scan is another useful tool. Whenever you're about to stand while holding your baby, pause and check: are your feet placed flat, knees over ankles, hips level, ribcage stacked over your hips? Are shoulders relaxed? Neck long, chin parallel to the ground? You don't need to fix everything at once. Just pick one thing to focus on each time. With repetition, these quick assessments become second nature, even when you're tired.

Tuning in to these small details isn't just about easing aches. It builds awareness of what feels good and what needs to change. Sometimes shifting your weight or relaxing your jaw releases tension immediately. You'll notice which chairs make you slouch and how holding baby on one side strains your neck. That awareness lets you make changes before discomfort sets in.

Improving posture isn't about perfection. It's about gradually feeling better. Even when progress is slow or inconsistent, every posture check is a small act of self-care showing you value your own comfort alongside your baby's needs. Over time, these small habits accumulate, transforming the way you sit, move, and rest each day.

You've learned to sit better, hold better, and move through feeds without wrecking your neck and shoulders. But what happens when you stand up? Picking your baby up off the floor, hauling the car seat, climbing stairs while carrying everything at once. Hack 6 is about protecting your back and core through all of it.

HACK 6: FUNCTIONAL LIFTING

"Exercise won't change the way you move. You have to change the way you move, and that can improve how muscles function."
—Dr. Shirley Sahrmann, PT, PhD, Washington University School of Medicine

You will lift your baby somewhere between 50 and 100 times per day. From the floor, the crib, the car seat, your own lap. Most of those lifts happen on autopilot, and that's exactly when your back pays the price. The overlooked truth is that how you lift your baby day after day affects your recovery just as much as any workout.

Your glutes are not just for gym squats. They stabilize your pelvis and protect your spine during lifting and carrying. Squeezing your glutes at the right moment shifts the effort away from your back and arms, turning each baby pick-up into a form of self-support. Strong glutes also help realign your hips, counteracting the changes from pregnancy and hours spent rocking or feeding. If you're dealing with diastasis recti or pelvic floor weakness, glute activation provides extra support, taking pressure off your core *(Reiman et al., 2012; Michaud et al., 2021).*

The Glute Squeeze Pick-Up: Protecting Your Back While Lifting Baby

The Glute Squeeze pick-up works from any surface. Whether you're lifting from a crib, floor, or playmat, the steps stay the same:

1. Place your feet hip-width apart, heels rooted firmly to the ground.

2. Hinge at your hips by pushing them back, like closing a car door with your backside. Let your knees bend just enough to lower toward your baby without rounding your back.

3. Keep your chest lifted and eyes forward as you reach down. Never twist sideways or lunge at an angle.

4. Gently brace your core, as if zipping up a snug pair of jeans.

5. As you stand to lift, squeeze your glutes and drive the movement through your hips. Keep it firm and controlled, not forceful.

6. Hold your baby close to your body. Don't let them drift away from your center as you rise.

Visual cues help, especially when you're tired: chest lifted, hips back, glutes squeezing. For the crib, keep your hips behind you and your shoulders relaxed, not hunched. From the floor, move slowly and with control. If your spine rounds or your chest collapses, pause, reset, and start again.

A common mistake is relying too much on arms and back, especially when rushed. You might find yourself lifting with rounded shoulders, straightening your legs first, or holding your breath. All of these strain healing muscles. When you catch yourself doing it, stop, reset your form, and try again.

Before using this move with your baby, especially early in recovery, practice with something light: a pillow, folded blanket, or a small basket. Run through the full movement three to five times a day. Use a mirror for feedback. Watching yourself can reveal hidden habits like slouching or tilting sideways.

Glute Squeeze Self-Check

After each practice, check in with yourself:

- Did your glutes activate at the top of the lift?

- Was your chest lifted and your back straight?

- Did you keep your baby or object close to your body?

Jot down what felt strong and where you felt shaky. Notice when your lower back feels better or when you feel more stable during daily lifts. Perfect form isn't realistic every time. The goal is awareness and repetition until the motion becomes second nature.

Car Seat and Stroller Lifting Modifications for C-Section Recovery

After a C-section, even everyday tasks like lifting car seats and strollers can feel overwhelming. The ache at your incision and general fatigue make heavy, awkward objects particularly difficult. The issue isn't just the weight; it's the angles and reaching motions that can provoke scar sensitivity or sudden pain. Those warning twinges aren't weakness. They are your body telling you it's still healing.

When you need to lift a car seat with your baby inside, break the movement into smaller steps:

1. Slide the seat as close to your body as possible before lifting anything.

2. If it's on the back seat, use both hands to scoot it toward you. Pivot your whole body, hips and feet included, rather than twisting at the waist.

3. Once it's close, pause and take a breath.

4. Bend your knees, keep your back upright, hands under the handle,

elbows hugged in.

5. Use your legs to lift. Work both legs and arms together rather than pulling with your core alone.

For strollers, set up your space before you lift. Open doors, clear pathways, and bring the stroller as close to your shins as possible. Grip with both hands, palms facing each other, and keep your wrists straight. If you need to turn, pivot your whole body rather than twisting at the torso. A gentle rocking motion can often free jammed or stuck gear more easily than a single hard heave.

Split-load strategies are especially helpful during this stage. Carry fewer items at a time, even if it means extra trips. With heavier strollers, try rolling or walking them out of the trunk instead of lifting. If needed, drag items toward you using a towel as a handle before lifting.

Whenever possible, slide rather than lift. Move car seats or strollers along a bench or seat before picking them up. For trunks, rest one end of the stroller on the bumper before lifting the rest inside. This small shift takes significant pressure off your healing body.

Don't hesitate to ask for help. This is not the time to prove your independence. Most people are happy to assist when asked clearly. Try: "I'm recovering from surgery. Could you help with the stroller?" or "Would you mind grabbing the car seat?"

If your budget allows, lightweight strollers or car seat caddies with rolling bases and cushioned handles make a real difference. Borrowing from friends works just as well for a short recovery window.

Quick Self-Check: How Does That Lift Feel?

After modifying any lifting strategy, pause for a moment:

- Is there pulling or sharpness near your incision or pelvic floor?

- Do you feel stable, or are you compensating with one side?

- If something feels wrong, make a note. Tracking discomfort helps you spot patterns and prevent injury.

This phase is temporary. Gentle movements, smart adjustments, and frequent help will serve you far better than toughing it out.

Core Engagement in Real Life: Laundry Baskets, Grocery Bags, and More

The first time you lug a laundry basket up the stairs or hoist a bag of groceries onto the counter with a baby on your hip, your body makes it very clear that things have changed. These tasks don't wait for the perfect moment. They happen when the dryer buzzes, when someone drops off groceries, or when your toddler needs a snack right now. In those moments, your core and pelvic floor should work for you, not against you.

Before you lift anything, even a basket of towels or a bulky diaper pail, take a breath out and gently draw your belly in, like zipping up a pair of jeans. Pair this with a gentle glute squeeze and you create a natural shield for your back and pelvis. Let your hips push back rather than bending at the waist. Keep your chest proud, gaze ahead, and maintain a neutral spine from head to tailbone. These small adjustments protect healing tissue and prevent the aches that build up through the day.

Household chores offer endless opportunities to practice. Before grabbing a laundry basket, place your feet hip-width apart. Exhale, set your core and glutes, hinge at your hips, and lift with the load held close to your body. If the basket is heavy, use both hands and hug it to your torso. Switch arms halfway through a trip to balance muscle fatigue. When moving grocery bags from the car, carry them close to your center rather than dangling at arm's length. If you need to grab something at an awkward angle, pause and pivot your whole body rather than twisting at the waist.

Before lifting bins, diaper pails, or pet food, do a quick check: Am I bracing my core? Are my shoulders relaxed? Am I about to round my back or twist? These questions become automatic with repetition. Sticky notes on the washing machine or fridge can help until they do. If you're especially fatigued, run through the movement empty-handed once before adding weight. This builds muscle memory so that even on autopilot, your body remembers how to move safely.

Fatigue is a real risk factor for injury. When your baby is wailing or dinner is burning, it's easy to forget good form entirely. Make it a habit to slow down for one breath and reset before any lift. Two trips with lighter bags are always better than one overloaded haul that leaves you sore.

At-Home Lifting Scenarios: Core Support Quick-Reference

- **Laundry baskets:** Plant feet hip-width apart; exhale and set core; hinge at hips; hug basket close; avoid twisting.

- **Grocery bags:** Carry bags close; alternate arms; keep elbows tucked; check posture before each lift.

- **Diaper pails and bins:** Use both hands; stand close; bend knees slightly; keep back tall.

- **Pet food and heavy toys:** Get as close as possible; use squat instead of bending at waist; pivot whole body if changing direction.

- **Tidying heavy toys/gear:** Kneel if needed, keep weight near center; avoid reaching far.

With every well-aligned lift, you're protecting yourself now and building a foundation for stronger days ahead.

Mini-Milestone Tracker: Noticing Less Pain and More Strength

Progress in the fourth trimester rarely looks like anything you'd track on a fitness app. It shows up in small, real-world moments you notice when you least expect them. Maybe your back doesn't ache after carrying your baby upstairs, or you lift a heavy bag without needing to pause halfway. These are the signposts that your micro-adjustments are paying off, even when it doesn't feel that way.

Try using a simple tracker, a checklist or a running note on your phone. Mark down any time a task feels easier than it did last week. Did you move the car seat without wincing? Were you able to buckle your baby in without holding your breath? Each of those moments counts. Over time, patterns emerge. Maybe after a weekend of rest you feel more confident in your movements, or Mondays are harder than Fridays. Noticing these rhythms helps you work with your body rather than against it.

Progress is the goal, not perfection. Some days you'll feel like you're back at square one, especially after a rough night or during a growth spurt when everything feels heavier. Other days the shift is small but real: less soreness after laundry day, an easier reach for a dropped pacifier. Those subtle wins matter. They're proof that muscle memory is building.

Journaling can help you spot these wins and reflect on your growth. At the end of the week, take five minutes and jot down answers to these questions:

- What was the easiest lift I did this week?

- Where did I feel unexpectedly strong?

- Did any movement trigger discomfort or make me pause?

Plateaus and setbacks are normal. Everyone hits them, especially when tired or juggling more than usual. If pain returns or something that felt easy suddenly feels hard again, pause and review what's changed. Are you more tired, stressed, or skipping those small self-checks? Sometimes pulling back to lighter loads for a few days is all it takes to get back on track. If new symptoms appear, sharp pain, persistent soreness, or weakness that doesn't fade, reach out to a pelvic floor physical therapist. Sometimes one session is all you need for reassurance and a clear path forward.

Consistency is what builds real change. Even slow progress, made with intention, adds up. Many moms are surprised by how much more capable they feel after just a couple of weeks of mindful lifting and tracking, even when sleep is still a mess and life feels chaotic.

Reflection Prompt: Celebrate Your Mini-Milestones

Take a moment to think about your week. Was there a task, no matter how small, that felt easier? Maybe you hefted the diaper bag into the car with less effort, or noticed less tension in your back after cooking dinner while baby-wearing. Write it down, circle it on your tracker, or just say it out loud. Your body is adapting, even when you doubt it.

You've built a real foundation now: breath, pelvic floor, posture, and the lifts that fill your day. In Hack 7, we shift our focus to keeping your body moving even when energy is low and time is short, simple routines that blend into daily life because healing happens in the in-between moments too.

HACK 7: STROLLER POWER

"Diaphragmatic breathing in the immediate postpartum period is the most underrated exercise that every woman should be focusing on. Instead of rushing back into jogging or running, allow your body to rest, heal and focus on building up your foundation."
—Dr. Heather Smith, PT, DPT, Pelvic Floor Physical Therapist, Hinge Health

Formula feeding meant I did not have the built-in excuse to sit down every two hours. My son took a bottle, my husband could do the feeds, and everyone around me seemed to think that meant I was somehow more available for normal life again. I was not. My body was still healing, still aching, still figuring itself out. The stroller became the one thing that made sense, not a workout or a goal, just forward motion and fifteen minutes of fresh air where the only job was to walk outside and come back a little more like myself.

Stroller Strides: Safe Walking Form to Support Core Recovery

Getting outside with your baby, even for ten minutes, can feel like reclaiming a piece of yourself during the exhausting early months of motherhood. When basic self-care feels impossible, a walk offers both a mental lift and real support for your body's healing. Research shows that as little as 15 minutes of walking a day can produce clinically significant reductions in postpartum depression symptoms *(Pentland et al., 2021)*. The key is intention. Every stroll can gently aid core and pelvic floor recovery when you walk with awareness, not just distance.

Walking form starts at your hands. When you grip the stroller handle, keep your wrists neutral, not angled up or down. Bend your elbows softly, as if hugging the handle rather than leaning over it. Before you set off, roll your shoulders up, back, and down to release tension. At crosswalks or curbs, consciously drop your shoulders and shake out your arms.

Good posture matters more than speed. Here are the key form cues to carry with you on every walk:

1. Stack your ears directly above your shoulders and hips. This tall alignment activates your core naturally and keeps your spine safe.

2. Keep your chest open. Breathe into your ribs as you move, not shallow at your chest.

3. As you exhale, gently draw your lower belly in, as if zipping up a pair of jeans. This is your core activation cue. No straining or sucking in, just a light gathering of your deep muscles.

4. Walk with even steps, landing softly through the center of your heel and rolling forward onto your toes.

5. Keep your strides short. A shorter step reduces pulling in your lower belly and pelvic pressure.

6. If your baby is fussy and you feel the urge to rush, consciously slow down to protect your form.

Start with five to ten minutes at a comfortable pace. If you feel well, add a minute or two every few days. Your tissues may still be healing even when you feel fine.

If you notice pelvic heaviness, sharp pain, or sudden fatigue, pause and rest. Listening to your body protects your long-term strength *(Pentland et al., 2021)*.

A few things to avoid: overstriding can worsen diastasis or cause pelvic pain. Slumping over the stroller handle might feel easier when you're tired, but it strains your back and core over time. Urinary leaking, pelvic heaviness, or new pain during a walk are all signals to slow down and check in with a pelvic floor physical therapist if symptoms persist.

Walking Form Checklist

Scan through these before and during your walk:

- Are my wrists straight and elbows soft?

- Are my shoulders dropped and relaxed?

- Is my head stacked over my hips?

- Am I stepping evenly and not overreaching?

- Do I feel my core gently activate with each exhale?

- Am I breathing fully into my ribs?

If any answer is no, pause and adjust before moving on.

With these small adjustments, stroller walks can become more than just a way to get fresh air—they are an accessible tool for real recovery, fitting seamlessly into your busy life as a new mom.

Five-Minute Stroller Stretch Routine

You don't need a studio or mat for relief. Your stroller handle becomes a simple support for stretches that release tension, restore flexibility, and gently wake up muscles strained by long nights and lifting. After my second baby, getting on the floor wasn't realistic. So instead I built a standing five-minute routine I could do anywhere: a sidewalk, a park, the pediatrician's parking lot. If you can stand and reach the stroller handle, you're ready.

Chest Opener

1. Place your hands wide on the stroller handle, arms outstretched.

2. Step your feet back slightly and lean forward just enough to feel a gentle stretch across your collarbones and shoulders.

3. Take three slow breaths, expanding your chest on each inhale and releasing tension on each exhale.

Hip Flexor Stretch

1. Hold the stroller handle for balance and step one foot back into a staggered stance.

2. Bend your front knee slightly and let your hips shift forward until you feel a stretch at the front of your back hip and thigh.

3. Hold for two to three breaths, then switch legs. If you had a C-section, keep the shift gentle. A small movement is enough.

Upper Back Release

1. Stand facing the stroller with hands on the handle, shoulder-width apart.

2. Soften your knees and push your hips back, folding gently forward from your waist with a flat back.

3. Let your head drop between your arms and feel the stretch from your

tailbone to the crown of your head. Hold for three slow breaths.

Calf Stretch

1. Stand behind the stroller and step one foot back, toes pointing forward.

2. Press your back heel firmly into the ground and lean gently forward into the stroller handle.

3. Hold for a count of ten, feeling the pull along your calf. Switch sides.

If your baby needs movement during any of these stretches, add gentle calf raises or slow knee bends as you hold the handle. A small push back and forth on the stroller soothes your baby and keeps you moving at the same time.

All these stretches are done standing or leaning—no need to get on the ground, making them easy and public-friendly, whether at a park, sidewalk, or even indoors during long days at home.

Save this list in your phone or slip it into your diaper bag for quick reference. With regular use these four stretches can become a natural bookend to any walk.

Micro-Mobility Hacks for Park Benches and Play Dates

Fitting movement into a busy mom's life doesn't require special gear or a workout window. Park benches, playground curbs, and low steps are perfect for gentle mobility work. While your baby naps in the stroller or plays nearby, you can ease tight hips, wake up your glutes, and release back tension without anyone noticing.

Seated Figure-Four Hip Stretch

1. Sit tall on the bench and cross your right ankle over your left knee.

2. Let your right knee relax open and lean forward slightly with a straight

back.

3. Hold for a few breaths, feeling the stretch in your hip and glute. Switch sides.

Bench-Supported Lunge

1. Stand beside the bench and place both hands on its edge for balance.

2. Step one foot back and gently sink your hips forward, keeping your front knee over your ankle.

3. Hold for a few breaths, feeling the stretch in your hip flexors and thighs. Switch sides.

Standing Twist

1. Stand beside the bench and rest one hand lightly on the back for support.

2. Sit tall through your spine and gently rotate your torso toward the bench.

3. Breathe into the stretch for two to three breaths, then rotate to the other side.

Moving in public can feel awkward at first, but most people are focused on their own children or conversations. If you feel self-conscious, just smile and carry on. Many moms will recognize what you're doing and may even join you.

Build movement into your park visit naturally. While your baby naps in the stroller, cycle through two stretches every ten minutes. If you're pushing a swing, alternate between calf stretches and standing side reaches. Tie movement to your existing routines: after buckling your baby in, sneak in a hip opener; after snack time, do a quick shoulder roll.

If you're recovering from a C-section or have joint discomfort, keep all movements slow and within a comfortable range. Avoid deep twists if you feel pulling near your scar. For a sensitive pelvic floor, stick to seated moves with both feet grounded. When time is short, pick just one stretch and repeat on each side while keeping an eye on your baby. Even a minute of intentional movement makes a difference.

Park Bench Mobility: Quick Reference

- **Seated Figure-Four:** Cross ankle over opposite knee, lean gently forward.

- **Bench-Supported Lunge:** Hands on bench, one foot back, hips forward.

- **Standing Twist:** One hand on bench, gently rotate torso.

- **Shoulder Rolls:** Sit or stand tall, roll shoulders up, back, and down.

- **Ankle Circles:** Seated, lift one foot and slowly circle the ankle.

Keep this list on your stroller or in your phone for those moments when you need quick inspiration. The body responds to repetition more than intensity. A two-minute stretch done five days in a row does more for your recovery than a perfect thirty-minute session once a week. Over time these brief resets become part of how you move through the day, not something you have to carve out time for. That's exactly how lasting recovery is built!

Seven hacks in, and something has quietly shifted. Maybe you noticed it the first time you caught yourself breathing properly during a feed instead of holding your breath through the exhaustion. Maybe it was the moment you picked up your baby from the floor and felt your body actually support the movement instead of bracing against it. Or maybe you just feel a little more like yourself than you did a few weeks ago, and you are not entirely sure why.

That is the work landing. It does not always announce itself loudly. Sometimes recovery looks like a slightly better morning, a walk that felt easier than the last one, a body that is slowly, quietly finding its way back. You showed up for yourself seven times when it would have been completely understandable not to, and that matters more than you probably realize right now.

What comes next is the other half of that same care. Because a body that is learning to move again also needs to be genuinely fed. Not just fueled with whatever is within reach, but actually nourished in a way that supports everything your body is working so hard to do. Part II is where that happens, and it was written for exactly the season you are in right now.

Every Mom Deserves to Know This

"If you have some power, then your job is to empower somebody else."
—Toni Morrison

Around three weeks after I had my son, my mother called to check in. I told her I had just done my pelvic floor exercises for the first time since coming home from the hospital. There was a pause, and then she laughed. Not unkindly. She just said, "I didn't even know that was a thing."

That conversation stayed with me for a long time. My mother had five children. She loved us fiercely, managed all of our schedules largely on her own, and never once had anyone walk her through what was happening to her body after each birth or what she could do about it. She just got on with it, the way her mother had, and her mother before that.

The exercises in Part I exist because that cycle deserves to be broken. Because you deserve to understand what is happening inside your body after birth and to have practical, honest tools to help it recover. Nobody should have to figure this out alone, and nobody should have to stumble across this information by accident years later.

If any part of Part I has helped you feel more connected to your recovery, I would love to ask one small favor. Leave a review on Amazon. It takes about as long as one set of the 360° Breath, and it puts this book in front of another mom who may not even know yet that this kind of support exists. Your experience is worth sharing.

[QR CODE **PLACEHOLDER**]

Now turn the page, because the second half of this book is where we make sure the body doing all that hard physical work is actually being fed.

PART II: NOURISHING RECOVERY

____

6 HACKS

FOUNDATION: FUELING THE FOURTH TRIMESTER

"Several nutrients contribute to our mental health before, during, and after pregnancy. Some of these include vitamins B2, B6, selenium, DHA, and zinc."
—Ryann Kipping, Prenatal Nutritionist and Founder of The Prenatal Nutrition Library

The first weeks after my baby arrived, my family filled my fridge. Dishes appeared on the counter without me asking, things that were warm and nourishing, the kind of food that felt like care. I was grateful, and I ate what was there. But even with all of that, something was still off. My energy was not returning the way I expected. My body felt like it was working against me rather than with me, and I could not understand why. I was eating. I was resting when I could. I was doing everything I thought I was supposed to do. And still, I felt depleted in a way I could not name or explain.

At the time, I blamed my body. I told myself I was not trying hard enough, not sleeping enough, not being disciplined enough. I assumed the problem was me, not the information I had never been given. Welcome to the club, by the way! Millions of members, zero meetings, and not one of us got the handbook. Later, I understood I was depleted, not just from birth, but from weeks of inadequate nourishment, mounting anxiety, and the quiet weight of postpartum depression

I had not yet named. I thought the anxiety and low mood were hormonal, driven by broken sleep and the sheer weight of adjustment. And those things were real. But I was also chronically underfed, and nobody had warned me that what I was eating, or not eating, was shaping how I felt every single day.

Whether you are breastfeeding, formula feeding, or combining both, your body is doing extraordinary work. It needs to be fed consistently and with intention, not perfectly, not expensively, just regularly and with care. That is what Part II is about.

What Postpartum Depletion Actually Means

Pregnancy is one of the most nutritionally demanding experiences a human body can go through. For nine months, your body prioritized your baby's development above your own reserves. DHA, the omega-3 fatty acid critical for brain function and mood regulation, was steadily transferred to your baby's developing brain. Iron was redirected to support your baby's blood supply. Magnesium, essential for sleep, stress response, and nerve function, was drawn down with every trimester. By the time you gave birth, your nutritional reserves were already running low.

Then comes the recovery itself. Birth, whether vaginal or by C-section, involves significant blood loss and physical stress. If you are breastfeeding, your body continues to prioritize your baby's nutritional needs over your own, pulling from whatever reserves remain. If you are formula feeding, your body is still healing, still rebuilding tissue, still trying to rebalance hormones in the aftermath of one of the most profound physical events of your life.

Here is what postpartum depletion actually looks like in real life:

- Crying without knowing why, or feeling a flatness that doesn't lift

- Brain fog so thick you forget mid-sentence what you were saying

- Bone-deep fatigue that sleep alone doesn't seem to fix

- Anxiety that spikes unpredictably, often in quiet moments

- Mood crashes in the afternoon, irritability you can't explain

- Hair loss, brittle nails, skin that feels dull and depleted

These aren't just "normal" postpartum symptoms to push through. Many of them are signals that your body is running on empty. Deficiencies in iron, DHA, vitamin D, magnesium, and B vitamins have all been linked to higher rates of postpartum depression and anxiety *(Ellsworth-Bowers and Corwin, 2012)*. This doesn't mean food is a cure for postpartum mental health struggles. It means that nourishment is a foundation, and without that foundation, everything else becomes harder.

The good news is that small, intentional changes to what you eat can make a real difference. Not a complete overhaul. Not a meal plan that requires two hours in the kitchen. Just the right foods, at the right times, eaten consistently enough to begin rebuilding what pregnancy and birth depleted.

Nourishment vs. Dieting: Know the Difference

The pressure to "bounce back" after having a baby is everywhere. Social media, well-meaning comments, and a culture obsessed with postpartum weight loss can make it feel like your body is a problem to fix rather than a system to support. Let's be clear: the fourth trimester is not the time to diet. Restricting calories when your body is healing, potentially breastfeeding, and managing the hormonal aftermath of birth does more harm than good. It slows tissue repair, disrupts milk supply, worsens mood, and deepens the very depletion this section is designed to address.

Nourishment is the opposite of dieting. It is about eating enough, eating consistently, and choosing foods that give your body what it actually needs right now. This means more protein to rebuild tissue, more healthy fats to support brain function and hormone production, more iron-rich foods to replenish what birth took, and more water than you think you need, especially if you are breastfeeding.

Here is how to tell the difference between nourishing yourself and falling into diet culture thinking:

Signs you are nourishing

- Eating when you are hungry without guilt

- Choosing foods because they make you feel stronger, not smaller

- Drinking water consistently throughout the day

- Noticing your energy is more stable after eating

- Allowing yourself treats without spiraling into shame

Signs you may be falling into diet culture

- Skipping meals to "get back on track"

- Counting calories while breastfeeding or healing

- Feeling guilty after eating something that wasn't "healthy"

- Restricting food groups without medical guidance

- Comparing your postpartum body to images online

If you notice the red flags showing up, pause. This is not the season for restriction. Your body grew, sustained, and birthed a human being. It deserves fuel, not punishment. The hacks in Part II are built around this principle. They are practical, realistic, and designed for real life with a newborn, not for a nutrition plan that requires a perfectly stocked kitchen and two free hands.

What These Six Hacks Will Give You

The next six hacks are designed to meet you exactly where you are: exhausted, time-starved, possibly one-handed, and trying to take care of yourself while keeping a tiny human alive. No complicated meal plans. No expensive superfoods. No guilt. Just practical, evidence-based nutrition strategies that fit into the chaos of the fourth trimester.

Hack 8 – Why You Feel So Low: explores the direct link between postpartum mood and the specific nutrients your body is running low on, and the everyday foods that genuinely help restore them.

Hack 9 – Why You Can't Think Straight: looks at why brain fog and mental cloudiness are not just tiredness, and the key nutrients that feed your thinking brain when it needs it most.

Hack 10 – Why Your Body Won't Heal: covers the two nutrients most critical for tissue repair and blood rebuilding after birth, and how to get more of them into your day without complicated meals.

Hack 11 – Why You're Always Thirsty: goes beyond "drink more water" with an honest look at electrolytes, what your body is actually losing, and a hydration strategy that works in real postpartum life.

Hack 12 – Why You're Eating But Still Depleted: addresses the gap between eating and actually nourishing, with a simple framework, practical recipes, and honest guidance for breastfeeding moms on what actually supports milk production.

Hack 13 – Why Supplements Aren't Enough: cuts through a billion-dollar supplement industry to tell you what actually matters, what is being marketed to you, and how to spend your money wisely when your body is still rebuilding.

Your body did something extraordinary. The depletion you may be feeling right now is not weakness. It is evidence of how much you gave. Part II is about giving something back, because nourishment is not a luxury reserved for when things slow down. It is the foundation that makes everything else possible. In Hack 8, we begin with something most postpartum moms never hear: that the fog, the flatness, and the anxiety are not just hormones. They are also hunger, and that is entirely within your power to change.

HACK 8: WHY YOU FEEL SO LOW

"Every brain deserves and benefits from proper nourishment."
—Dr. Drew Ramsey, MD, Nutritional Psychiatrist, Columbia
University; Author of Eat to Beat Depression and Anxiety

Nobody warned me about the flatness.

Not the crying, everyone warns you about that. Not the exhaustion, that's practically a postpartum cliché at this point. I mean the specific, quiet heaviness that settles in somewhere around week two or three, when the newborn adrenaline starts to wear off and you realize you just feel... low. Not dramatically sad. Not obviously broken. Just muted, like someone turned the brightness down on everything, including you.

I assumed it was hormones. I assumed it was the broken sleep. And those things were real. I was dealing with postpartum anxiety and the beginning of depression, and I won't pretend food was the only answer, because it wasn't. But what nobody told me was that my brain was also running on empty in a way that had nothing to do with how hard I was trying or how much I loved my baby. It was running low on the raw materials it needed to regulate my mood. And I had no idea.

What Pregnancy Did to Your Brain

Here is something most doctors don't mention at your six-week checkup: by the time you gave birth, your brain had already been quietly depleted for months.

During pregnancy, your body made a series of decisions on your baby's behalf, and one of the most significant was this. When DHA became limited, your body prioritized your baby's developing brain over yours. DHA, short for docosahexaenoic acid, is the fatty acid that forms roughly 30 percent of your brain's gray matter — the part responsible for memory, emotions, and decision-making. Think of it as your brain's structural foundation. When it runs low, everything from mood regulation to mental clarity starts to feel off. Your body didn't take it from you carelessly. It did what it was designed to do. But it leaves your brain working with less of what it needs to keep you feeling stable, clear, and calm.

At the same time, magnesium, a mineral involved in producing serotonin, regulating cortisol, and keeping your nervous system from staying permanently on edge, was steadily drawn down throughout pregnancy. The fetus and placenta take what they need. By the time you are holding your baby, many women are already running a deficit they don't know about, and the stress of new motherhood pulls that deficit deeper with every passing week.

Then there is vitamin D. Your brain has vitamin D receptors in the exact regions responsible for mood regulation, the hippocampus, the hypothalamus, and the prefrontal cortex. When vitamin D is low, neuroinflammation increases and the production of mood-regulating neurotransmitters is disrupted. Research has found a consistent link between lower vitamin D levels in the postpartum period and higher rates of postpartum depression *(Aghajafari et al., 2018)*. And in the early weeks of new motherhood, getting outside for even fifteen minutes of sunlight feels like something that happens to other people.

None of this is your fault. Your body protected your baby the way it was designed to. Now it needs you to return the favor.

What Traditional Wisdom Gets Right, and Where It Gets Honest

In many Asian cultures, the weeks after birth are treated as a period of intentional recovery. Families cook. Mothers rest. Specific foods are prepared with care, not because someone read a nutrition label, but because generations of women passed down what helped them feel stronger, recover faster, and feed their babies well.

Some of these traditions have real nutritional backing that modern research has since confirmed. Bone broth, simmered slowly from marrow-rich bones, delivers collagen, glycine, and minerals that support tissue repair and gut health. Moringa, used across Southeast Asia and parts of Africa for centuries, is genuinely one of the most nutrient-dense foods available, rich in iron, calcium, B vitamins, and compounds that support milk production. Warming soups made with ginger, sesame, and black chicken are not just comfort food. They are recovery food, built from centuries of women paying attention to what their bodies needed.

But here is the honest part.

My family made winter melon soup in the early weeks after I gave birth. Also called wax gourd, it is one of the most traditional galactagogue foods in Chinese postpartum culture, believed to help mothers produce more breast milk. I ate it faithfully and gratefully. And it did not help me. My milk supply stayed low regardless, and no amount of winter melon changed that.

This doesn't mean the tradition is wrong. It means bodies are individual. Galactagogues, foods believed to support milk production, work beautifully for some women and have no measurable effect on others. Whether you are breastfeeding, formula feeding, or combining both, your nutritional needs in the postpartum period are significant and real. This hack isn't about prescribing one food or promising one fix. It is about understanding what your body is actually missing and finding sustainable, realistic ways to start filling those gaps, in a way that works for your body and your life.

The Foods That Actually Help

You don't need a meal plan. You don't need to overhaul your kitchen or source expensive ingredients. What you need is to understand which foods do the most work with the least effort, and find small, repeatable ways to include them.

For Mood and DHA:

- **Fatty fish:** salmon, sardines, mackerel, and anchovies are the richest sources of EPA and DHA. Aim for two to three servings a week.

- **Walnuts, chia seeds, and flaxseeds:** good plant-based options that your body partially converts to DHA. Easy to add to oatmeal, yogurt, or smoothies.

- **Algae-based omega-3 supplements:** the most direct plant-based source of DHA, worth discussing with your provider especially if you are not eating fish regularly.

For Magnesium and Nervous System Calm:

- **Pumpkin seeds:** one of the richest magnesium sources available, no preparation needed. A small handful as a snack or sprinkled on top of anything counts.

- **Dark chocolate, at least 70 percent cacao:** provides magnesium alongside brain-supporting flavonoids. A square or two is enough.

- **Almonds, cashews, spinach, black beans, and edamame:** reliable everyday sources that fit into real postpartum eating without needing a recipe.

For Vitamin D:

- **Fatty fish:** covers both DHA and vitamin D at once, which is why it tops every list in this hack.

- **Egg yolks:** one of the most useful postpartum foods overall, delivering vitamin D, protein, choline, B12, and healthy fat in three minutes flat.

- **Fortified plant milks and orange juice:** smaller amounts, but every bit adds up.

- **Sunlight:** even ten to fifteen minutes of direct sun during a stroller walk supports vitamin D production in a way no supplement fully replicates.

For Gut Health and Serotonin:

About 95 percent of your serotonin is produced in your gut, not your brain. A recent study found that postpartum mothers with lower gut microbiota diversity had significantly higher depression scores, and that eating fermented foods was one of the most consistent dietary factors linked to better mood outcomes *(Matsunaga et al., 2025)*. One serving of something fermented daily is enough to start supporting a healthier gut environment. Pick one below and make it a habit.

- **Yogurt with live cultures:** the most accessible option; choose plain, full-fat varieties

- **Kefir:** drinkable and easy to grab with one hand

- **Kimchi or sauerkraut:** alongside any meal, even just a spoonful counts

- **Miso:** stirred into warm water as a savory drink between feeds

- **Kombucha:** lower sugar varieties for a lighter option

Try This Tonight

Before you do anything else, pick one of these. Just one. Each takes under three minutes and requires one hand.

- **The Mood Bowl:** Full-fat plain yogurt, a handful of walnuts or pumpkin seeds, a drizzle of honey. Probiotics, DHA precursors, magnesium, and protein in one bowl.

- **The Sardine Toast:** Whole grain toast, a tin of sardines in olive oil, a squeeze of lemon. Rich in DHA, vitamin D, calcium, and B12. Keep a few tins in the cupboard for the days when cooking feels impossible. This is one of those meals that asks almost nothing of you and gives a lot back.

- **The Miso Moment:** A teaspoon of miso paste stirred into a mug of warm water. Sip it between feeds. Thirty seconds, one hand, and a meaningful dose of beneficial bacteria for your gut.

None of these are perfect meals. They are intentional moments, small acts of nourishing yourself in the middle of everything else. That is, honestly, exactly enough.

Reflection Prompt: Check In with Yourself

- Have you eaten anything today that wasn't grabbed out of necessity?

- When did you last eat something that felt like it was actually for you?

- Of the foods mentioned in this hack, which one could you realistically add this week?

Write it down, note it in your phone, or just sit with it for a moment. You don't have to change everything. You just have to start somewhere.

The flatness you feel is not a character flaw. It is not proof that you are failing. It is your depleted brain asking for something specific, and now you know what that something is. Hack 9 takes this further, into the brain fog, the forgetfulness, and the feeling that your mind belongs to someone else. Because what you eat shapes not just how you feel, but how clearly you can think.

HACK 9: WHY YOU CAN'T THINK STRAIGHT

"The brain is not a static organ. It changes in response to experience, and motherhood is one of the most powerful experiences it will ever navigate"
—Dr. Elseline Hoekzema, Neuroscientist, Leiden University; Maternal Brain Study

My friend Sofia had her baby three weeks before mine. Sofia grew up in a Mexican-American household where food was how you showed up for people, and postpartum recovery was a family affair, full stop. When she was discharged from the hospital, her mother had already driven six hours from San Antonio and taken over the kitchen. She arrived with two bags of dried chiles, a slow cooker, and approximately forty years of opinions about postpartum recovery. The house filled up quickly, mother, mother-in-law, a cousin, a neighbor who somehow also came, and for the next three weeks, Sofia was fed constantly, bathed in advice, and lovingly managed by women who knew exactly what a new mother needed. She was grateful. She told me later that she spent those weeks smiling and nodding while quietly losing her mind. "Everyone was doing everything," she said. "But I couldn't get a single quiet moment to think. And I still couldn't remember words."

My experience was different but somehow identical. When I had my baby, my family arrived with containers of congee, black sesame soup, and firm instructions that I was not to wash my hair for thirty days. This is a traditional Chinese postpartum practice rooted in the belief that the body loses significant heat during birth, and that exposing yourself to cold, including cold water, slows recovery and invites illness. Modern medicine doesn't fully support the hair-washing rule, but the instinct behind it is real: your body after birth is vulnerable, depleted, and in need of warmth and protection. I nodded along. I also secretly rinsed my hair on day four and told nobody.

Then there was Amy, another friend of mine. American, practical, loving, and completely on her own. Her parents had both passed away, and she and her husband lived two states away from his family. When the baby came, there was no one to call. Her husband went back to work after two weeks. And so Amy, six weeks postpartum, was doing the grocery runs, the laundry, the night feeds, and the dishes largely by herself. She had no one telling her what to eat or when to rest. She also had no one to hand the baby to when she needed ten minutes to feel human again. "I just thought this was how it worked," she told me. "I thought everyone felt this way."

Three women. Three completely different postpartum experiences. One shared reality: none of us could finish a sentence, all of us kept losing things, and every single one of us thought something was wrong with us personally.

Nothing was wrong with us. Our brains were running low on the raw materials they needed to function. And nobody had told us that what we ate, or didn't eat, in those early weeks was directly shaping how clearly we could think.

Your Brain Didn't Break. It Renovated.

Here is the part that genuinely changes how you see yourself during this season.

During pregnancy, your brain undergoes a process that neuroscientists have only recently begun to document. Gray matter, the part of the brain responsible for processing information and forming memories, reduces slightly in regions associated with social cognition. When researchers first observed this in brain imaging studies, they assumed it was damage. Further investigation revealed something completely different. The reduction is deliberate. Your brain was pruning away less essential neural connections to make room for something more important: an extraordinary sensitivity to your baby's needs, cues, and emotional state *(Hoekzema et al., 2017)*.

Think of it the way a skilled gardener thins a plant, not to weaken it, but to direct its energy toward what matters most. Your brain became more efficient at reading your baby's face, distinguishing their cry from every other sound in the world, and anticipating what they need before they can communicate it. That is not cognitive decline. That is cognitive specialization, and it is remarkable.

The fog you are feeling is the side effect of a brain that gave everything to this reorganization and then ran out of the raw materials it needed to complete the rebuild. It is not broken. It is just underfueled.

The Two Nutrients Your Brain Is Missing Most

While DHA plays a major role in mood as we covered in Hack 8, two other nutrients have the most direct impact on the sharpness, speed, and clarity of your thinking: choline and iron. Both are depleted significantly by pregnancy and birth. Both are rarely discussed at postpartum checkups. And both make a measurable, documented difference when they are restored.

Choline and the Memory Gap

Choline is an essential nutrient that your body uses to produce acetylcholine, the neurotransmitter directly responsible for memory, attention, and learning. Think of acetylcholine as the chemical messenger that carries a thought from one part of your brain to another. When it is abundant, information moves quickly and clearly. When it is low, thoughts feel slow, slippery, and hard to hold onto.

During pregnancy, your body's demand for choline increases dramatically as it supports fetal brain development. Most women don't consume enough choline to begin with. Studies show that the average woman gets only about 70 percent of her daily choline needs from food, and pregnancy depletes whatever reserves exist *(Zeisel, 2006)*. If you are breastfeeding, the drain continues after birth because breast milk is rich in choline for your baby's still-developing brain.

The result shows up as the specific kind of forgetfulness that feels almost embarrassing: walking into rooms and forgetting why, losing words mid-sentence, reading the same paragraph three times and retaining nothing. This is not sleep deprivation alone. It is a choline gap, and it is entirely addressable through food.

Iron and the Processing Slowdown

Iron deficiency is one of the most common consequences of childbirth, and one of the least discussed in terms of its cognitive effects. Research has found a strong and direct relationship between iron status and cognitive functioning in postpartum women. In one landmark study, iron-deficient mothers showed significantly slower processing speed, reduced accuracy across cognitive tasks, and higher rates of depression and stress compared to iron-sufficient mothers. When iron levels were restored, cognitive performance improved by 25 percent *(Beard et al., 2005)*.

Iron is the mineral your brain uses to synthesize dopamine and serotonin, the two neurotransmitters most associated with motivation, focus, and mood. When iron is low, your brain cannot produce these chemicals efficiently. The result is a sluggishness that goes beyond physical tiredness: a mental slowness that makes even simple decisions feel effortful, and that no amount of sleep seems to fix.

Here is what most moms don't know: you can be low in iron without being anemic. Standard postpartum bloodwork checks hemoglobin levels, but iron deficiency can affect cognitive function well before anemia shows up on a test. If you feel mentally sluggish but your doctor says your blood work looks fine, it is worth asking specifically about your ferritin levels, which reflect your iron stores rather than just your red blood cell count.

The Foods That Feed Your Thinking Brain

You don't need a supplement stack or a complex meal plan. You need a handful of specific foods that your brain genuinely responds to, eaten consistently enough to begin rebuilding what pregnancy and birth depleted.

For Choline

- **Eggs:** the single most bioavailable source of choline available, with one whole egg providing roughly 147mg. The yolk is the important part, so don't skip it.

- **Salmon:** provides both choline and DHA in one serving, making it one of the most efficient postpartum brain foods available.

- **Chicken liver or chicken liver pate:** a small serving delivers more choline than almost any other food. Pate on whole grain toast is an accessible and surprisingly good starting point.

- **Soybeans and edamame:** excellent plant-based choline sources, easy to grab from the freezer and eat one-handed.

- **Full-fat dairy:** modest choline contributions that add up meaningfully across the day.

For Iron

- **Lean red meat:** provides heme iron, the most easily absorbed form available. Even a small serving two to three times a week makes a measurable difference.

- **Lentils and legumes:** excellent plant-based iron sources. Pair them with something vitamin C-rich, a squeeze of lemon, some tomatoes, or a splash of orange juice, to significantly increase absorption.

- **Pumpkin seeds:** portable, one-handed, and a reliable source of non-heme iron that fits easily into postpartum snacking.

- **Spinach:** pairs beautifully with eggs or legumes and provides both iron and folate, another nutrient critical for brain function.

- **Dark chocolate:** provides non-heme iron alongside magnesium and brain-supporting flavonoids. A square or two genuinely earns its place on this list.

One Pairing That Matters More Than You Think

Non-heme iron, the kind found in plants, absorbs far more effectively when eaten alongside vitamin C:

- A bowl of lentils with a squeeze of lemon.

- Spinach scrambled into eggs with a glass of orange juice.

- Black beans with a handful of cherry tomatoes.

- A handful of edamame with sliced kiwi on the side

- Pumpkin seeds stirred into a smoothie with frozen mango or strawberries

This single habit can dramatically increase how much iron your body actually uses from plant-based sources, without changing what you eat, just how you combine it.

Try This Tonight

Start with whichever one you already have ingredients for.

- **The Thinking Bowl:** A soft-boiled egg halved over warm brown rice, a handful of edamame, and a drizzle of soy sauce with a squeeze of lemon. Choline from the egg, plant-based iron from the edamame, vitamin C from the lemon to pull it all together. Five minutes, one hand, genuinely filling.

- **The Iron Hour:** A warm bowl of canned lentils with wilted spinach stirred through, topped with a spoonful of plain yogurt and a pinch of cumin. The vitamin C from the yogurt and the natural iron in the cumin work together quietly. One of the most nourishing postpartum meals you can make in under three minutes.

- **The Clarity Smoothie:** A frozen banana, a tablespoon of peanut butter, a handful of spinach, a cup of fortified plant milk, and a small square of dark chocolate blended together. Iron, choline precursors, magnesium, and enough sweetness to feel like a treat rather than a prescription.

Reflection Prompt: Check In with Your Clarity

- When did you last eat an egg, or any reliable source of choline?

- Are you pairing plant-based iron sources with something vitamin C-rich?

- On the days you feel sharper, what did you eat the day before?

That last question is worth sitting with. Most moms don't track the connection between food and mental clarity because the effect takes a day or two to show up. But it is there. And once you start noticing it, it becomes one of the most motivating things about eating well postpartum.

The fog lifts. It does, gradually and then more quickly than you expect. Your brain is not failing. It reorganized itself for you and your baby, and now it needs you to feed it back to strength. Hack 10 addresses the next piece of the picture: why your body feels slower to heal than you expected, and which specific nutrients make tissue repair happen faster than it would on its own.

HACK 10: WHY YOUR BODY WON'T HEAL

"The wound heals from the inside out. You cannot rush it. But you can feed it."
—Dr. Alejandro Junger, MD, Integrative Medicine Physician and
Author

About seven weeks after Amy's C-section, she called me. Not because anything was wrong, but because she needed to talk to someone who wouldn't tell her she was doing great. Her incision was still tender. Her energy was nowhere. She had just been cleared at her six-week checkup, handed a green light, and sent back into normal life. Grocery runs, laundry, a husband back at work, a baby who didn't care about any of it. "The doctor said everything looks good," she told me. "But I don't feel good. I feel like my body is still figuring out how to be a body again."

She mentioned she had gone for a walk at two weeks postpartum just to get out of the house, and had spent the whole time feeling guilty for not doing more. I laughed and told her that in Chinese postpartum tradition, the expectation is the complete opposite. For the first thirty days, new mothers are supposed to rest so completely that even reading and watching too much television is discouraged, because it strains the eyes and depletes the body's recovering energy. Leaving the house is off limits. Lifting anything heavier than your baby is off limits. The whole

91

philosophy is built around one idea: your body just did something extraordinary, and now it needs everything you have to rebuild.

Amy went quiet for a second. Then she said, "Wait. So I've been feeling guilty for not doing enough, and you've been feeling guilty for doing too much?" We laughed for a good minute on that call.

But underneath the laughter was something neither of us had fully named yet. We were both still depleted. Amy's incision was healing slowly. My energy had never quite come back the way I expected. And the real reason wasn't just that we needed more rest or more time. It was that our bodies were trying to repair themselves without the specific raw materials they needed to do it. Rest matters. Time matters. But healing is also a matter of nutrition, and that is the part nobody puts in the discharge paperwork.

The Six-Week Clearance Is a Starting Line, Not a Finish Line

Here is something worth knowing about your postpartum body that most six-week checkups don't cover: the biological process of healing continues long after a doctor clears you for normal activity.

Whether you had a vaginal birth with tearing, an episiotomy, or a C-section, your body is working through three distinct phases of wound repair: inflammation, tissue rebuilding, and remodeling. The remodeling phase alone, where collagen fibers reorganize and strengthen, can continue for up to a year after birth. A C-section involves healing through seven layers of tissue. Perineal tears require sustained amino acid supply for proper recovery. And inside the uterus, where the placenta was attached, there is a wound roughly the size of a dinner plate that needs to close, rebuild, and strengthen from the inside out *(Marshall et al., 2022)*.

The six-week clearance reflects what is visible and measurable at a brief clinical appointment. It does not reflect the full picture of what your body is still doing beneath the surface. And if your diet is not providing what the healing process requires, that process slows down in ways that show up as persistent tenderness, fatigue that doesn't improve, and a general sense that your body is just not quite right.

The Two Things Your Body Is Building With

Physical healing after birth is not a passive process. It requires raw materials, specifically protein and vitamin C, working together to rebuild the tissue that pregnancy and birth disrupted.

Protein: The Foundation of Every Repair

Protein is not just for muscle building. It is the structural material your body uses to rebuild skin, connective tissue, the uterine wall, and everything else that needs to be restored after birth. The amino acids glycine, proline, and lysine are the specific building blocks your body needs to produce collagen, the protein that forms the structural scaffold of healing tissue *(Shoulders and Raines, 2009)*.

Research shows that protein needs increase significantly during all phases of wound healing, with some studies suggesting requirements rise by up to 250 percent compared to baseline. For a C-section recovery in particular, where the body is healing through multiple layers of tissue simultaneously, adequate protein intake is one of the most direct things you can do to support the process. Most postpartum women are eating far less protein than their healing bodies actually need, often because appetite is suppressed, meals are rushed, and nobody told them this was a priority.

Vitamin C: The Collagen Activator

Vitamin C is the essential cofactor that activates the enzymes your body needs to build and stabilize collagen. Without adequate vitamin C, collagen synthesis is compromised and tissue heals more slowly, more weakly, and with a greater tendency toward complications. Research confirms that vitamin C levels drop significantly at wound sites immediately after injury, and that adequate intake is associated with faster healing, stronger tissue, and reduced scarring *(Carr and Maggini, 2017)*.

The connection between vitamin C and postpartum recovery is direct. Your incision, your perineal tissue, your uterine wall: all of them are producing collagen right now. And every one of those processes depends on vitamin C to proceed properly. The traditional postpartum foods that appear across cultures, warming broths, ginger soups, nutrient-dense stews, are not random. They are, in many cases, foods that provide exactly the amino acids and micronutrients that tissue repair requires. The science caught up to the tradition eventually.

The Foods That Actually Rebuild You

Your body is already running the repair process around the clock. What determines how well it goes is whether the right materials are arriving consistently enough to keep up with the demand.

For Protein and Collagen Building Blocks

- **Bone broth:** if someone offers to cook for you, this is what to ask for. Rich in glycine, proline, and collagen precursors, it is one of the most restorative postpartum foods across cultures. Store-bought versions work just as well for daily use.

- **Lean beef or lamb:** a small serving two to three times a week provides complete protein, zinc, and iron together, all three of which directly support tissue repair and blood rebuilding.

- **Chicken thighs:** more forgiving than breast meat, stay moist when reheated, and freeze well. Cook a batch when you have help and pull from it throughout the week.

- **Tofu and tempeh:** plant-based complete protein that absorbs whatever flavor you cook it in. Add to soups, stir fries, or eat straight from the packet on the days when cooking isn't happening.

- **Cottage cheese:** underrated, genuinely high in protein, and one of the easiest one-handed postpartum foods available. Eat it plain or topped with fruit straight from the container.

For Vitamin C and Collagen Activation

- **Bell peppers:** richer in vitamin C than most citrus fruits. Slice a few at the start of the week and keep them in the fridge as an instant grab-and-go option.

- **Kiwi fruit:** two kiwis exceed your entire daily vitamin C requirement. No preparation, no cooking, fits in one hand.

- **Papaya:** one of the highest vitamin C fruits available and often overlooked. Also contains natural digestive enzymes that help a postpartum gut absorb nutrients more effectively.

- **Broccoli:** steamed into soups or stir fries rather than raw makes the nutrients more bioavailable and easier on a postpartum digestive system.

- **Mango:** easy to eat one-handed, generous in both vitamin C and vitamin A, and sweet enough to feel like a treat rather than a nutritional obligation.

The Pairing That Makes It Work

Protein and vitamin C are most effective when they appear in the same meal:

- Bone broth with a side of sliced kiwi or bell pepper

- Cottage cheese topped with mango and a drizzle of honey

- Chicken thigh and broccoli stirred through warm rice

- Tofu and papaya in a simple warm broth

- Lean beef strips with sliced bell pepper over noodles

This combination is not a nutrition strategy. It is simply what warming, restorative postpartum cooking looks like across most food traditions in the world. Your grandmother probably knew this even if she couldn't explain the biochemistry.

Try This Tonight

Your body is already working hard. Make this the easy part.

- **The Rebuild Bowl:** Warm bone broth poured over cooked rice or noodles with shredded rotisserie chicken and sliced bell pepper on top. Protein, collagen precursors, vitamin C, and carbohydrates in one bowl. Ten minutes, one hand, genuinely nourishing.

- **The Healing Plate:** Cottage cheese in a bowl topped with sliced mango, a drizzle of honey, and a small handful of sunflower seeds. High protein, vitamin C, and healthy fat in two minutes flat.

- **The Recovery Broth:** A mug of warm store-bought bone broth with a handful of frozen broccoli dropped in and a squeeze of lemon. Collagen precursors, vitamin C, and minerals in three minutes. Ask someone to keep your freezer stocked with this.

Reflection Prompt: Check In with Your Recovery

- Are you eating any source of protein at every meal, including breakfast?

- When did you last eat something rich in vitamin C?

- Is your body healing at the pace you expected, and if not, what has your nutrition looked like this week?

Healing is not just a waiting game. It is an active process that your body is running in the background every hour of every day, whether you are feeding it properly or not. The difference is in how well and how quickly that process can do its job. You have more influence over that than you might think.

Your body is not failing at healing. It is healing as well as it can with what it has been given. The more consistently you give it what it actually needs, the more you will feel the difference. Hack 11 addresses the next piece of the picture: *why you are always thirsty*, why water alone is not enough, and what your body is actually asking for when it sends you to the kitchen for the fourth time in an hour.

HACK 11: WHY YOU'RE ALWAYS THIRSTY

"Water is the driving force of all nature."

—Leonardo da Vinci

There is a specific kind of thirst that hits at the exact moment your baby latches. Not a gentle suggestion to drink something. A sudden, fierce, almost desperate need for water that arrives like a wave and does not let up until you have drained whatever is within reach. If you have experienced this, you are not imagining it. It is built into the biology of breastfeeding. The moment your baby begins feeding, oxytocin releases to trigger milk letdown, and your hypothalamus responds by triggering thirst at the same time. Your body is telling you, in no uncertain terms, that what is leaving needs to be replaced immediately.

But here is what most new moms don't realize until they are deep in the fog of it: replacing fluid is not the same as replacing what your body is actually losing. Breast milk is roughly 90 percent water, and every feed pulls not just fluid but electrolytes, minerals, and nutrients directly from your body. When you are formula feeding, your body is still recovering from birth, still rebalancing hormones, still healing. The dehydration of the postpartum period is not just about water. It is about everything that water carries with it.

Why "Drink More Water" Is Incomplete Advice

Eight glasses of water a day is advice designed for a resting, non-lactating adult who slept last night. It was not designed for someone producing up to 700 to 800 milliliters of fluid daily through breastfeeding, healing from birth, running on broken sleep, and sweating through postpartum night sweats.

Research confirms that exclusively breastfeeding mothers consistently end their days with a fluid deficit, even when they believe they have been drinking enough. In one study, breastfeeding mothers were found to have the lowest daily water balance of any population studied, with an average daily deficit of around 475 milliliters despite conscious efforts to stay hydrated *(Tziatzios et al., 2024)*. The problem is not willpower or forgetfulness. The problem is that plain water, consumed in isolation, does not stay in your cells the way water consumed alongside electrolytes does.

Electrolytes, which include sodium, potassium, magnesium, calcium, and chloride, are the minerals that regulate how your body absorbs and retains fluid. When electrolyte levels are low, water passes through your system without being properly absorbed. You can drink glass after glass and still feel parched, foggy, and depleted. That specific combination of constant thirst alongside persistent fatigue, muscle cramps, and headaches is not a hydration problem alone. It is an electrolyte gap, and plain water cannot fill it.

What Your Body Is Actually Losing

Every feed transfers electrolytes from your body into your milk. Breast milk contains measurable concentrations of sodium, potassium, and chloride that are drawn directly from maternal stores *(Semba and Juul, 1997)*. Beyond breastfeeding, postpartum night sweats, one of the most common and least discussed postpartum experiences, deplete sodium and potassium further every night. And the stress of sleep deprivation elevates cortisol, which disrupts the kidneys' ability to retain electrolytes efficiently.

The result is a slow but steady depletion that shows up as:

- Persistent thirst that water alone does not satisfy

- Afternoon headaches with no obvious cause

- Muscle cramps, particularly in the legs at night

- A foggy, disconnected feeling that is different from ordinary tiredness

- Sluggish milk letdown or a sense that supply has dipped without explanation

None of these are inevitable. They are signals that your electrolyte balance is off and that your hydration strategy needs more than a bigger water bottle.

What Actually Hydrates You

The most effective postpartum hydration comes from a combination of fluids and electrolyte-rich foods that your body can absorb and use at the cellular level.

Electrolyte-Rich Drinks

- **Coconut water:** a natural source of potassium and sodium with no added sugar. One cup provides a meaningful electrolyte contribution alongside genuine hydration. Keep it in the fridge and reach for it during feeds.

- **Warm herbal broths:** clear vegetable or miso broth provides sodium and trace minerals in a warm, soothing format that also supports digestion. Particularly useful during night feeds when cold drinks feel jarring.

- **Homemade electrolyte water:** a pinch of sea salt and a squeeze of citrus in a large glass of water. The sodium supports fluid absorption; the citrus adds potassium and vitamin C. Simple, free, and genuinely effective.

- **Whole milk or fortified plant milk:** provides fluid alongside calcium, potassium, and protein, making it one of the most nutritionally complete hydration options for postpartum recovery.

Hydrating Foods That Also Replenish Minerals

- **Cucumber:** about 96 percent water, with natural silica that supports connective tissue. Slice it and keep it in the fridge for immediate access throughout the day.

- **Watermelon:** high water content alongside potassium and natural sugars that support electrolyte absorption. Easy to eat one-handed in chunks.

- **Banana:** one of the most reliable potassium sources available, easy to eat during a feed, and provides natural carbohydrates that support energy and electrolyte balance simultaneously.

- **Avocado:** rich in potassium and healthy fats that support hormone production and slow the depletion of electrolytes. Half an avocado on anything counts.

- **Sweet potato:** provides potassium alongside complex carbohydrates and vitamin A. Bake a batch when someone offers to help and eat from it throughout the week.

The Breastfeeding Thirst Strategy

Rather than trying to track how much you are drinking, anchor your hydration to your feeding rhythm. Every time your baby feeds, you drink. Not a sip. A full glass. This habit alone, practiced consistently, brings most breastfeeding mothers close to their actual fluid needs without counting a single cup.

For formula feeding moms, the same principle applies differently: anchor your drinking to moments that already exist in your day. Every nappy change, every time you sit down, every alarm on your phone. The goal is not a number. It is a consistent rhythm that replaces what your body is quietly losing throughout the day.

And when you feel that desperate wave of thirst hit, honor it. Your hypothalamus is doing its job. Reach for something with electrolytes, not just plain water, and notice the difference in how quickly the thirst actually resolves.

Try This Tonight

Pick whichever feels most doable right now.

- **The Feed Drink:** Fill a large glass with cold water, add a pinch of sea salt and a squeeze of lemon or orange. Keep it next to wherever you feed. Drink the whole glass during one feed tonight. Simple, effective, and one of the most consistent hydration habits postpartum moms report actually sticking to.

- **The Night Replenisher:** A warm mug of miso or vegetable broth beside your bed for night feeds. Sodium, minerals, and warmth in thirty seconds. Ask whoever is helping to set it up before bed.

- **The Morning Reset:** A cup of coconut water with half a banana alongside whatever you normally eat for breakfast. Potassium, natural sodium, and fluid together before the day depletes you further.

Bonus: Your Free Postpartum Hydration Tracker

Knowing what to drink is one thing. Actually remembering to drink it when you are in the middle of a feed, a nappy change, and a baby who will not settle is another thing entirely. That is why I created a free printable Postpartum Hydration

Tracker you can download, print, and keep wherever you spend most of your time with your baby.

The tracker includes a simple daily checklist to help you build the feed-and-drink rhythm from this hack into your actual day. Scan the QR code below to download your free printable Postpartum Hydration Tracker.

Download it, print it, and tape it somewhere you will actually see it during feeds. Your future self will thank you.

Reflection Prompt: Check In with Your Hydration

- Does your thirst feel satisfied after drinking water, or does it linger even when you have had plenty?

- Are you experiencing afternoon headaches, leg cramps, or a foggy disconnection that feels different from ordinary tiredness?

- What is the easiest moment in your current daily rhythm to anchor a consistent drink?

The best hydration strategy is the one that fits into what is already happening in your day. Not a perfect system. Not a new habit built from scratch. Just one consistent moment, repeated often enough to make a difference.

Thirst is one of the body's most honest signals. When it persists despite drinking, it is pointing at something specific. Now you know what that something is. Hack 12 moves into the part of postpartum nutrition that ties everything together: the meals, the system, and the recipes that make nourishing yourself within reach when you are exhausted, one-handed, and running on the kind of sleep that barely counts as sleep.

HACK 12: WHY YOU'RE EATING BUT STILL DEPLETED

"So many people end up depleted after pregnancy and birth. And it doesn't matter if you give birth vaginally or via C-section, there's depletion."
—Lucy Chapin, CNM, NP, Certified Nurse Midwife, Peripartum Nutrition Specialist

A certified nurse midwife named Lucy Chapin, who specializes in peripartum nutrition, wasn't talking about moms who weren't eating. She was talking about moms who were eating constantly, grabbing whatever was nearest, surviving on whatever was nearest, whatever required zero effort, and still ending up more depleted than when they started.

That was me. And based on every conversation I have had with other moms, it was probably you too.

I wasn't skipping meals. I was eating throughout the day. But what I was eating, the granola bar grabbed on the way to the fridge, the toast I made at 7am and ate cold at noon, the spoonful of peanut butter standing at the counter, was filling the gap without filling the tank. My body was running on the nutritional equivalent of spare change. Enough to keep going. Not enough to actually recover.

Research confirms that most postpartum women fail to meet recommended intake for key nutrients including vitamin D, iron, folate, and omega-3 fatty acids, not because they aren't eating, but because what they are eating in survival mode doesn't come close to covering what their healing, hormonal, and potentially lactating bodies actually need *(Sebastiani et al., 2024)*. The problem isn't appetite. It isn't even access. It is the invisible gap between eating and nourishing, between filling your stomach and actually feeding your recovery.

This hack closes that gap.

The Difference Between Eating and Nourishing

Survival eating has a very specific pattern. It happens fast, with one hand, standing up, between one task and the next. It reaches for whatever requires the least decision-making. It prioritizes volume over quality because hunger is immediate and cooking is not. And it leaves you fed but somehow still empty, because the foods that fill you fastest, crackers, processed snacks, refined carbohydrates, are also the ones that spike and crash your blood sugar, provide minimal micronutrients, and burn through your system before the next feed.

The postpartum body needs significantly more than maintenance calories. It needs specific nutrients to repair tissue, regulate hormones, stabilize mood, and if breastfeeding, produce milk that nourishes a growing baby. When those nutrients are consistently missing, the depletion that began in pregnancy deepens. You eat, but your reserves don't rebuild. You sleep when you can, but the fatigue doesn't lift. You do everything you're supposed to and still feel like something is wrong.

Nothing is wrong. The system is just missing a few critical inputs.

The Five-Minute Postpartum Plate

The solution is not a meal plan. Meal plans require planning, and planning requires mental bandwidth that new motherhood does not leave available. The solution is a framework, a simple, flexible way of building a meal in under five minutes from whatever is already in the house.

Every time you eat, aim for three things together:

Something that fills and fuels: a complex carbohydrate that releases energy slowly and keeps blood sugar stable. Oats, quinoa, sweet potato, brown rice, or whole grain toast. Oats deserve special mention here. They are one of the most widely consumed and traditionally recognized foods for supporting breastfeeding, rich in iron, beta-glucan fiber, and compounds that may support milk production *(Ryan et al., 2023)*. A bowl of oats is genuinely one of the most postpartum-appropriate meals you can eat.

Something that rebuilds: a protein source that provides the amino acids your body needs for tissue repair, hormone production, and sustained energy. Nut butter, hummus, cheese, canned fish, a handful of seeds, leftover meat, canned chickpeas. It does not need to be a full portion or a perfectly balanced meal. It just needs to be present.

Something with color: a fruit or vegetable that adds vitamins, minerals, and antioxidants. A handful of berries on your oats. Sliced fruit on the side. Frozen vegetables stirred into whatever you are warming up. The color is the signal that micronutrients are present, and micronutrients are what survival eating consistently misses.

Three elements. Five minutes. No recipe required.

The Breastfeeding Plate

If you are breastfeeding, your body has additional nutritional needs beyond general recovery. Producing milk requires approximately 330 to 400 extra calories per day, along with increased demand for protein, calcium, iodine, choline, and specific compounds that support milk production itself. This section is specifically for breastfeeding moms. If you are formula feeding, the Five-Minute Postpartum Plate fully covers your needs and you can move straight to the recipes below.

The Truth about galactagogues

Every postpartum food tradition in the world has its version of milk-supporting foods. Chinese mothers eat black sesame preparations and warming soups. Indian mothers eat dal and fenugreek. Filipino and African mothers eat moringa. Korean mothers eat miyeok-guk, a seaweed soup, within hours of giving birth. American lactation consultants recommend oats and brewer's yeast. These traditions exist because women across centuries noticed what helped. Here is what the current evidence actually shows:

- **Moringa** has the strongest research backing of any food galactagogue. A systematic review of eight clinical trials found that moringa supplementation increased breast milk volume by up to 400 milliliters per day compared to controls, with meaningful effects on prolactin levels *(Bettinelli et al., 2025)*. Add moringa powder to smoothies, soups, or warm drinks.

- **Oats** are the most widely used food galactagogue among breastfeeding mothers, with more than 40 percent of users reporting perceived increases in supply. The mechanism is thought to relate to their iron content and beta-glucan fiber, though large-scale clinical evidence is still limited *(Ryan et al., 2023)*.

- **Brewer's yeast** is high in B vitamins, iron, and protein, and is frequently reported as effective by breastfeeding mothers. It has a strong taste on its own but blends almost undetectably into oatmeal, smoothies, or lactation cookies where it is masked by other flavors.

- **Fenugreek** is one of the most widely known herbal galactagogues worldwide, but the evidence is genuinely mixed. Some studies show meaningful increases in milk volume. Others show no effect. A smaller number of women report it actually decreasing supply. If you try it, monitor your supply carefully and discontinue if things worsen.

- **Fennel and sesame seeds** appear across multiple traditional postpartum food cultures and provide meaningful nutritional support regardless of their effect on supply. Add fennel to warm teas or soups. Sprinkle sesame seeds or tahini on anything.

The most important thing to understand about galactagogues is that no food or supplement creates supply that is not there. The primary drivers of milk production are frequent, effective milk removal and adequate overall nourishment. These foods support the conditions that make good milk production possible. They are not magic, but they are genuinely useful, and for many moms they make a real difference.

A Note on Measurements

If you have read through Part II this far, you may have noticed that the measurements here look a little different from what you would find in a standard cookbook. No weighing. No precise fractions. No standing over a measuring cup with a leveling knife while the baby decides that right now is the perfect time to need you. Where a quantity genuinely matters for a recipe to work, you will find simple guides like a cup, a teaspoon, or enough to fill the jar halfway. Where it does not matter, you will find a handful, a drizzle, or a generous spoonful. Trust yourself! Cooking in the fourth trimester is not about precision. It is about getting something nourishing into your body with whatever you have and however much time you actually have!

Feed Yourself First

These twenty recipes below are built for real postpartum life. No precise measurements, no complicated steps, no ingredients you need to make a special trip for. Each one follows the three-element framework: something filling, something rebuilding, something with color. Mix and match, repeat what works, and ignore what doesn't.

Breakfast

The Overnight Jar

- Rolled oats, enough to fill the jar halfway

- Oat milk, poured in until it just covers the oats

- A spoonful of nut butter

- A handful of berries

Seal and refrigerate the night before. Grab straight from the fridge in the morning, no reheating! This jar is powerful in carbohydrates, protein, healthy fat, and antioxidants before you even think about what day it is.

The Golden Porridge

- Rolled oats, enough to fill a mug or bowl halfway

- Hot water or oat milk, about twice the volume of the oats

- A pinch of turmeric

- A pinch of ginger

- A drizzle of honey

- A sprinkle of sesame seeds

Stir oats into the hot liquid and cook for three to five minutes until thick and creamy. Stir through spices and honey. Top with sesame seeds. Anti-inflammatory and genuinely comforting at any hour.

The Savory Rice Bowl

- Warm leftover brown rice

- One egg

- A drizzle of soy sauce

- A handful of frozen edamame, thawed

Fry the egg and lay it over the warm rice. Drizzle soy sauce and add edamame alongside. Yes, rice for breakfast. Warm, filling, protein-forward, and done in four minutes.

The Amaranth Porridge

- Amaranth, enough to fill the bottom third of a small pot

- Coconut milk, about two and a half times the volume of the amaranth

- A handful of chopped dates

- A sprinkle of toasted sesame seeds

Simmer amaranth in coconut milk, stirring occasionally, until thick and creamy, about fifteen to twenty minutes. Top with dates and sesame seeds. Complete protein, iron, and natural sweetness in one bowl.

The Hemp Seed Smoothie Bowl

- Two large handfuls of frozen berries

- A small splash of oat milk, just enough to get the blender moving

- A generous sprinkle of hemp seeds

- A drizzle of tahini

- A few sliced dates

Blend berries with the smallest amount of oat milk needed to blend smoothly. You want thick, not pourable. Pour into a bowl and top with hemp seeds, tahini, and dates. Complete protein, omega-3s, and magnesium in forty-five seconds.

Snacks

The Date and Tahini Stack

- Two or three Medjool dates

- A small spoonful of tahini per date

Split dates open and press tahini inside each one. Iron, natural sugar, healthy fat, and calcium in thirty seconds. Keep a container of these ready in the fridge.

The Nori Roll-Up

- One sheet of roasted nori

- A spoonful of hummus

- A handful of brown rice or quinoa

Spread hummus on the nori, add the grain, and roll up. Fold in half and eat like a wrap. Iodine, protein, and carbohydrates. Genuinely one-handed once assembled.

The Trail Mix Jar

- Roasted chickpeas

- Sesame seeds

- Dried cranberries

- A few squares of dark chocolate, broken up

Mix everything in a jar. Make a big batch at the start of the week and eat from it throughout. No preparation required at the point of eating.

The Flaxseed Yogurt Cup

- Plain yogurt

- A generous spoonful of ground flaxseed

- A handful of berries

- A drizzle of honey

Stir flaxseed through the yogurt, add berries and honey on top. Omega-3s and fiber with no change to taste or texture. Two minutes, one hand.

The Nut Butter Rice Cake Tower

- Two rice cakes

- A thick layer of almond or peanut butter

- Banana slices

- A dusting of cinnamon

Stack and eat one-handed. Carbohydrates, protein, healthy fat, and potassium in ninety seconds.

Quick Meals

The Quinoa Power Bowl

- Warm pre-cooked quinoa

- A handful of frozen vegetables, microwaved

- A spoonful of tahini

- A squeeze of lemon

Combine and eat. Rotate the vegetables every time so it never gets repetitive. Complete protein, minerals, and healthy fat in four minutes.

The Chickpea Stir Bowl

- One tin of chickpeas, drained

- A drizzle of olive oil

- A pinch of cumin

- A pinch of turmeric

- Salt to taste

- Brown rice or whole grain bread to serve

Warm chickpeas in a pan with olive oil and spices for three minutes. Serve over brown rice or with bread. Iron, protein, and fiber in under five minutes.

The Tuna Wrap

- One tin of canned tuna, drained

- A spoonful of hummus

- A squeeze of lemon

- Fresh or dried herbs if available

- A whole grain tortilla

Mix tuna with hummus and lemon, roll into the tortilla. Eat in one hand. Protein, healthy fat, and B12 in three minutes.

The Miso Noodle Soup

- Noodles of any kind, a generous handful

- Two cups of water or light broth

- One heaped teaspoon of miso paste, stirred in off the heat

- A handful of frozen vegetables

- A soft-boiled egg, halved (optional)

Cook noodles in water or broth, drop in frozen vegetables in the last two minutes. Remove from heat before stirring in miso so the good bacteria survive. Top with egg if available. Warming, mineral-rich, and done in eight minutes.

The Sheet Pan Sweet Potato and Chickpea Bake

- One medium sweet potato, cubed

- One tin of chickpeas, drained

- A drizzle of olive oil to coat

- A good pinch of cumin and salt

Toss everything together, spread on a tray in a single layer, and roast at 400 degrees for 25 minutes until golden. Produces three to four servings. Ask someone to set this up before they leave. You just eat from it all day.

The Ginger Carrot Soup

- Four to five medium carrots, roughly chopped

- A thumb-sized piece of fresh ginger

- Three cups of vegetable broth

- A pinch of turmeric

Simmer everything together for twenty minutes until carrots are completely soft. Blend smooth. Thin with a little extra broth if needed. Make a large pot when you have help, freeze in individual portions, and reheat in a mug.

No-Cook Options

The Hummus Plate

- Hummus

- Vegetables or crackers, whatever is within reach

This is not a recipe. It is a permission slip to call hummus and crackers a meal when that is what the day allows. Protein, iron, fiber, and healthy fat without a single minute of cooking.

The Date Energy Ball

- Six to eight Medjool dates, pitted and mashed

- A handful of rolled oats, roughly equal in volume to the mashed dates

- A spoonful of nut butter

- A sprinkle of sesame seeds

Mix everything together until it holds when pressed. If too sticky, add a few more oats. If too dry, add another spoonful of nut butter. Roll into balls and refrigerate. Make a batch once a week.

The Overnight Oat Jar Remix

- Rolled oats, enough to fill the jar halfway

- Your choice of milk, poured in until it just covers the oats

- A small spoonful of chia seeds

- A spoonful of nut butter

- Whatever fruit is nearby

Assemble in a jar the night before. The oats will absorb the milk overnight and swell to fill the jar. Eat cold straight from the jar in the morning. No heating, no bowl required.

The Seaweed and Avocado Wrap

- One sheet of roasted nori

- Half an avocado, mashed

- A pinch of sea salt

- A handful of leftover grain

Spread avocado on the nori, add grain and salt. Roll up and eat immediately. Iodine, healthy fat, potassium, and carbohydrates in two minutes with zero heat.

The Breastfeeding Kitchen

These fifteen recipes below were created with breastfeeding moms in mind, built around the galactagogue foods and broader nutritional demands that come with making milk. That said, if you are formula feeding and any of this appeal to you, go ahead. Calcium, iron, iodine, and anti-inflammatory support are not exclusive to breastfeeding bodies. The first eight recipes feature galactagogue ingredients with the strongest evidence and traditional backing. The final seven focus on broader nourishment, including calcium, iodine, iron, and anti-inflammatory support. All of them follow the same principle: **genuinely nourishing and genuinely doable.**

Galactagogue Recipes

The Classic Lactation Oatmeal

- Rolled oats, enough to fill a bowl halfway

- Oat milk, about twice the volume of the oats

- One teaspoon of brewer's yeast

- A spoonful of almond butter

- A handful of berries

Cook oats in oat milk over medium heat for three to five minutes, stirring until thick and creamy. Stir in brewer's yeast, top with almond butter and berries. The brewer's yeast is almost completely masked. The most widely used galactagogue combination for a reason.

The Moringa Green Smoothie

- One frozen banana

- One teaspoon of moringa powder

- A spoonful of almond butter

- One cup of oat milk

- A drizzle of honey

- A large handful of frozen mango

Blend everything together until completely smooth, about sixty seconds. Add a little more oat milk if needed to blend. Moringa has the strongest research backing of any food galactagogue. The mango and honey completely mask the earthy flavor.

The Fennel Tea Latte

- One teaspoon of fennel seeds

- One cup of hot water

- Half a cup of warm oat milk

- A drizzle of honey

Steep fennel seeds in hot water for five minutes, strain into a mug. Top with warm oat milk and honey. One teaspoon is enough. More than that tips from pleasantly anise-flavored into overpowering. Particularly good during night feeds.

The Sesame Tahini Energy Balls

- One cup of rolled oats

- Three tablespoons of tahini

- One teaspoon of brewer's yeast

- One teaspoon of molasses

- Two tablespoons of ground flaxseed

- A drizzle of honey to bind

Mix everything together. The mixture should hold its shape when pressed. If too dry, add a little more honey or tahini. Roll into balls and refrigerate for at least thirty minutes before eating. Makes about ten to twelve balls.

The Lactation Overnight Oats

- Rolled oats, enough to fill the jar halfway

- Oat milk, enough to just cover the oats

- A splash of coconut milk for creaminess

- One teaspoon of ground flaxseed

- One teaspoon of brewer's yeast

- A small spoonful of chia seeds

- A handful of frozen berries

Layer everything in a jar, stir gently, seal and refrigerate overnight. The oats will absorb the liquid and the chia seeds will swell. Grab cold from the fridge in the morning. Four different galactagogue ingredients in one jar that requires zero morning effort.

The Moringa Golden Milk

- One cup of oat milk

- Half a teaspoon of moringa powder

- Half a teaspoon of turmeric

- A pinch of ginger

- A drizzle of honey

Warm oat milk in a mug, whisk in all ingredients until smooth. Sip during a feed. Two of the most evidence-backed postpartum support foods combined in one warm cup.

The Brewer's Yeast Banana Pancakes

One ripe banana, well mashed

- One cup of oat flour

- One teaspoon of brewer's yeast

- Oat milk, added gradually until batter pours like thick cream

Mix banana, flour, and brewer's yeast together. Add oat milk slowly until the batter is thick but pourable, not runny. Cook small stacks on a lightly oiled pan over medium heat until bubbles form, then flip. Freeze extras and reheat in thirty seconds. The banana completely masks the brewer's yeast.

The Fenugreek Lentil Dal

- One cup of red lentils, rinsed

- One small onion and two garlic cloves, diced

- Half a teaspoon of fenugreek seeds

- One teaspoon of cumin

- Three cups of vegetable broth

Soften onion and garlic in a little oil, add fenugreek and cumin and stir for one minute. Add lentils and broth, simmer for twenty to twenty-five minutes until lentils are completely soft and the dal is thick. Ask someone to make a large pot, portion into containers, and freeze for you. You just reheat from frozen.

Extra Nourishment Recipes

The Iodine Seaweed Broth

- One mug of vegetable or chicken broth

- A small piece of dried kombu seaweed

Warm broth in a mug, steep kombu for five minutes, remove and sip. Breastfeeding significantly increases iodine requirements. One of the simplest and most targeted breastfeeding drinks available.

The Hemp Seed Nourishment Bowl

- Warm pre-cooked quinoa

- A generous sprinkle of hemp seeds

- A drizzle of tahini

- Sliced dates

- A pinch of sea salt

Combine in a bowl and eat warm. Complete protein, omega-3s, magnesium, and iron in one bowl that takes three minutes to assemble.

The Calcium Power Smoothie

- One cup of oat milk

- A large handful of frozen mango

- A spoonful of tahini

- A small handful of kale

- A drizzle of honey (optional)

Blend until completely smooth. Add a little more oat milk if the blender struggles. Calcium from the oat milk and tahini, vitamin C from the mango to help absorb it, iron and folate from the kale.

The Nori Brown Rice Onigiri

- Cooked brown rice, still slightly warm

- Nori sheets, cut or torn into strips

- A pinch of sea salt

Wet your hands lightly, shape rice into small balls or triangles, press firmly so they hold. Wrap in nori and season with salt. Make several at once and keep in the fridge for up to three days. One-handed, portable, and rich in iodine.

The Turmeric Chickpea Warm Bowl

- One tin of chickpeas, drained

- A drizzle of olive oil

- Half a teaspoon of turmeric

- A pinch of ginger

- A squeeze of lemon

- Quinoa or whole grain bread to serve

Warm chickpeas in a pan with olive oil, turmeric, ginger, and lemon for five minutes. Serve over quinoa or with bread. Anti-inflammatory and high in plant-based iron.

The Molasses Oat Energy Bar

- Two cups of rolled oats

- Two tablespoons of molasses

- Three tablespoons of nut butter

- Two tablespoons of sesame seeds

- Two tablespoons of ground flaxseed

- A drizzle of honey to bind

Mix all ingredients together until evenly combined. The mixture should be sticky enough to press and hold. Press firmly into a lined dish about an inch thick. Refrigerate for at least two hours before slicing. Make once, eat all week. Molasses is one of the richest plant-based iron sources available.

The Coconut Millet Porridge

- Millet, enough to fill a small pot a quarter of the way

- Coconut milk, about three times the volume of the millet

- A generous sprinkle of hemp seeds

- Sliced dates

- A pinch of cinnamon

Simmer millet in coconut milk over medium-low heat, stirring regularly, for twenty to twenty-five minutes until thick and creamy. Top with hemp seeds, dates, and cinnamon. Millet is a traditional galactagogue across several West African postpartum food traditions, providing iron, magnesium, and B vitamins.

Reflection Prompt: Check In with What You're Actually Eating

- When you ate today, did what you ate contain at least one of the three elements: something filling, something rebuilding, something with color?

- Is there one simple swap you could make this week, replacing one survival food with one that actually nourishes?

- If you are breastfeeding, have you tried any of the galactagogue foods in this hack?

Small, repeatable, and within reach is always better than perfect and impossible. Your body is doing extraordinary work. Feed it accordingly.

Every hack in Part II has been building toward one truth: nourishing yourself postpartum does not require a perfect diet, an organized kitchen, or two free hands. It requires the right information and a system that fits into real life. Hack 13 covers the final piece, supplements, what actually matters, what is being marketed to you, and how to spend your money wisely when your body is still rebuilding.

HACK 13: WHY SUPPLEMENTS AREN'T ENOUGH

"Caring for myself is not self-indulgence. It is self-preservation."
—Audre Lorde

During pregnancy, I did everything my OB told me to do. I took my prenatal vitamin every morning without fail. I tracked what I ate, watched my caffeine, avoided the foods on the list, and showed up to every appointment. Nobody had to remind me. For the first time in my life, taking care of myself felt like taking care of someone else too.

Then my baby arrived, and somewhere in the blur of those first weeks, I stopped paying attention to what I was putting into my own body. Not intentionally. Not out of carelessness. But because the urgency I had felt for nine months quietly transferred the moment the baby was out. My job now was to take care of him. My own nutritional needs moved down the list without me even noticing.

I have spoken to enough moms to know this is not just my story. During pregnancy, we are the most motivated we will ever be to nourish ourselves. After birth, we become the least. And that is exactly when our bodies need the most support.

So let's talk about what that support actually looks like, what is worth your money, what is not, and how to make the smartest decisions for your body when your energy for decision-making is already running on empty.

Why Supplements Cannot Do What Food Does

Walk into any pharmacy, scroll through any parenting group, or spend five minutes on social media as a new mom and you will encounter the same overwhelming wall: supplements for energy, supplements for hair loss, supplements for milk supply, supplements for mood, supplements for skin, supplements for sleep. The postpartum supplement market is currently worth over one billion dollars and is projected to nearly double by 2032 *(Grand View Research, 2024)*. Every product promises to solve a problem you are very definitely experiencing. And when you are exhausted, depleted, and running on almost nothing, the idea that one capsule a day could fix the worst of it is genuinely appealing.

Some of those capsules are worth your money. Most are not.

The foundation of postpartum recovery is food. Real, nourishing, consistent food that gives your body the proteins, fats, carbohydrates, vitamins, and minerals it needs to heal, function, and if breastfeeding, produce milk. That is what the previous five hacks have been building toward. Supplements exist to fill gaps that food cannot reliably close on its own. They are not a replacement for eating well. A postnatal multivitamin taken alongside a day of crackers and survival snacks will not produce the same recovery as that same multivitamin taken alongside the nourishing meals in Hack 12.

There is also an important quality issue that most supplement marketing does not mention: up to 18 to 40 percent of commercially available prenatal and postnatal supplements contain undeclared pharmaceuticals, heavy metals, or incorrect dosages *(Keats et al., 2025)*. The supplement industry is not as tightly regulated as pharmaceutical drugs. This does not mean all supplements are unsafe. It means the brand and quality of what you buy genuinely matters, and that third-party tested supplements from reputable manufacturers are worth the extra cost.

The Supplements That Actually Matter

These are the nutrients with the strongest evidence for postpartum recovery. Not because someone is marketing them. Because research consistently shows that postpartum women are commonly deficient in these specific nutrients, and that deficiency has measurable consequences for how you feel, how you recover, and if breastfeeding, the nutritional quality of your milk.

Continue your prenatal vitamin, or switch to a postnatal

The simplest starting point: do not stop taking a multivitamin after birth. Your prenatal is an acceptable option to continue, though a dedicated postnatal formula is better calibrated to your needs after birth. Prenatal vitamins are formulated primarily for fetal development during pregnancy. Postnatal formulas generally provide more vitamin D, DHA, and choline, and in some cases better-calibrated iron. If you had a straightforward birth and your iron stores have recovered, continuing the higher iron doses designed for pregnancy may actually be more than your postpartum body currently needs *(InfantRisk Center, 2021)*. When in doubt, ask your provider.

Vitamin D

Vitamin D deficiency is one of the most common postpartum nutritional gaps, particularly for moms who gave birth in winter, live in northern climates, or spend most of their time indoors with a newborn, which describes most new moms at least some of the time. Research consistently links low vitamin D levels with increased risk of postpartum depression. A 2024 meta-analysis found that vitamin D deficiency was associated with significantly higher rates of postpartum depression in lactating women *(Yuan et al., 2024)*. The association is strong enough and the supplement inexpensive enough that most healthcare providers now recommend maintaining adequate vitamin D levels throughout the postpartum period. Look for vitamin D3, which is more bioavailable than D2.

DHA

DHA is the omega-3 fatty acid that forms the structural foundation of brain tissue. Maternal DHA stores can reduce by up to 50 percent during pregnancy and typically do not return to pre-pregnancy levels until around six months postpartum *(Innis, 2003)*. If you are breastfeeding, your baby's brain development is directly supported by the DHA concentration in your milk, which is determined by your own intake. Research shows that infants of mothers with higher breast milk DHA concentrations show improved brain and vision development outcomes. Many prenatal vitamins contain DHA but often in amounts below what is recommended. A separate omega-3 supplement providing at least 200 milligrams of DHA daily is commonly recommended for breastfeeding moms and remains a sensible choice for all postpartum women.

Iron

Blood loss during delivery is universal. Significant blood loss, which occurs in roughly one in five deliveries, can dramatically worsen iron stores that were already depleted during pregnancy. Iron deficiency is one of the most direct contributors to postpartum fatigue, brain fog, and mood instability, the very symptoms most commonly written off as just part of new motherhood. The World Health Organization recommends iron supplementation for the first six to twelve weeks postpartum. If you experienced heavy blood loss, ask your provider to check your ferritin levels at your postpartum visit and supplement accordingly. Note that if your iron stores have recovered and you are breastfeeding, your daily iron needs during lactation are actually lower than during pregnancy, around nine milligrams compared to twenty-seven, due to lactational amenorrhea reducing iron loss.

Iodine

Iodine is essential for thyroid hormone production, which regulates energy, metabolism, and mood. It is also critical for infant brain development and is actively secreted into breast milk, which means breastfeeding significantly increases a mother's iodine requirements. Yet iodine is one of the most consistently under-supplemented nutrients in postnatal formulas. The American College of Obstetricians and Gynecologists recommends 290 micrograms of iodine daily throughout the first year after birth. Check your prenatal or postnatal label specifically for iodine. Many formulas do not include it in adequate amounts, and many moms have no idea.

Choline

Choline is essential for brain function, liver health, and infant neurological development, yet it is consistently underrepresented in both diet and supplements. Postpartum women only met 39 percent of their choline requirements from food alone in one research review *(Keats et al., 2025)*. Breastfeeding increases choline requirements even further. Look for it specifically on your postnatal supplement label. If it is absent or present only in small amounts, consider a targeted supplement or prioritize choline-rich foods like eggs, which remain one of the most concentrated and accessible dietary choline sources available.

As with any supplement, always check with your healthcare provider before adding anything new to your routine, even over-the-counter vitamins. What your body needs depends on your birth experience, your current diet, and your individual health history. A quick conversation with your OB, midwife, or doctor is always the smartest first step.

What Is Being Marketed to You

The following supplements appear frequently in postpartum marketing. Some are genuinely useful in certain situations. Others are designed to solve problems that are more effectively addressed through food, rest, and the foundational supplements above.

Collagen

Collagen supports skin, hair, joints, and connective tissue. After birth, particularly after a C-section or significant tearing, collagen production matters for tissue repair. The most evidence-supported way to help your body produce collagen is through adequate vitamin C and protein, which support your body's own collagen synthesis. Supplemental collagen peptides are not harmful and may offer some benefit for skin and joint support, but the evidence is less robust than marketing suggests. If you enjoy collagen powder in your morning drink and it fits your budget, it is not a bad choice. Just do not prioritize it over the foundational supplements above.

Biotin

Biotin is heavily marketed for postpartum hair loss, which affects around 68 percent of new moms. Here is what the marketing does not tell you: postpartum hair loss is caused by hormonal shifts, specifically the drop in estrogen after birth, not biotin deficiency. Unless your biotin levels are actually low, supplementing will not prevent or significantly reverse the hair loss, which is temporary and resolves on its own within six to twelve months. Iron, zinc, and vitamin D are more directly connected to hair health. Address those first.

Probiotics

Probiotics support gut health, which can be genuinely disrupted after birth by hormonal changes, possible antibiotic use during labor, and the physical stress of delivery. Some research suggests specific strains may help with postpartum constipation and potentially mood, though the evidence for mood benefits is still emerging *(emerging research)*. If you experienced significant digestive disruption after birth or were given antibiotics during labor, a probiotic with evidence-backed strains is a reasonable addition. If your digestion is functioning well, the fermented foods from Hack 12 are a more affordable way to support your microbiome.

Energy and Sleep Supplements

Products marketed specifically for postpartum fatigue and sleep are a growing category. Some contain magnesium, which has evidence for supporting sleep quality and muscle recovery and is a reasonable addition to your routine. Others contain adaptogens, herbal compounds marketed for stress and energy, with variable evidence and limited postpartum-specific research. If fatigue is your primary concern, addressing iron, vitamin D, and hydration first is more likely to produce noticeable results than any adaptogen blend.

How to Choose What to Buy

The most common mistake in postpartum supplement shopping is buying too many products that duplicate each other. A postnatal multivitamin that already contains vitamin D, iron, iodine, and choline does not need four additional single-nutrient supplements alongside it unless your levels have been specifically tested and found to be deficient.

Start here and build only if needed:

- **One quality postnatal multivitamin.** Look for third-party tested, certified by NSF, USP, or an equivalent body. Look for methylated folate rather than folic acid, methylcobalamin rather than cyanocobalamin for B12, and iron bisglycinate rather than ferrous sulfate if iron is included. These forms are more bioavailable and gentler on digestion.

- **A separate DHA supplement.** Most postnatal vitamins do not include enough. Aim for at least 200 milligrams of DHA daily. Algae-based

DHA is the best option if you are fish-averse or prefer a plant-based source.

- **Vitamin D3 if not already in adequate amounts in your multivitamin.** Most postpartum women benefit from 1000 to 2000 IU daily. Ask your provider to test your levels if you are unsure.

- **Iron only if indicated.** Only if your ferritin levels are low or you experienced significant blood loss. Getting tested rather than supplementing blindly is always the smarter approach.

Everything else is optional, based on your specific symptoms, dietary gaps, and budget.

Before starting any new supplement, even one available over the counter, check with your healthcare provider first. Over-the-counter does not always mean appropriate for every body, and some nutrients interact with medications or have upper limits that matter during the postpartum period.

Try This Tonight

You do not need to overhaul anything tonight. Just do this one thing:

- Pick up your current supplement bottle and read the label.

- Does it contain iodine?

- Does it contain choline?

- Does it contain DHA in a meaningful amount?

Those three are the most commonly missing from standard postnatal formulas. If any are absent, that is exactly where your next supplement purchase should go.

Reflection Prompt: Know What Your Body Actually Needs

- Of the five foundational supplements covered in this hack, which ones are you currently taking?

- Are there symptoms you have been experiencing, fatigue, hair loss, brain fog, low mood, that might point to a specific deficiency worth investigating with your provider?

- Is there anything in your current supplement routine that duplicates what is already in your multivitamin?

Getting to the end of Part II means you have done something most new moms never get the chance to do: you stopped long enough to understand what your body has been going through and what it actually needs to recover. That is not a small thing. You came into this section exhausted, depleted, and probably surviving on whatever was within reach. You are leaving it with a framework for eating that works in real life, a clear picture of the nutrients your body is asking for, and the knowledge to make smarter decisions about what you spend your time and money on.

The six hacks in Part II were never designed to be a perfect plan. They were designed to meet you where you are, one meal, one supplement, one glass of water at a time. Some of what you read will become part of your daily rhythm quickly. Other pieces will take longer to find their place. Both are completely fine. Recovery is not a race and it does not follow a schedule.

What matters is that you showed up for yourself. In the middle of one of the most demanding seasons of your life, you chose to learn, to understand, and to nourish. That deserves to be recognized. Before we reach the Conclusion, I have one small favor to ask.

For the Sofia and Amy in Your Life

"We don't heal in isolation, but in community."

—S. Kelley Harrell

At some point during the writing of this book, I thought about Sofia sitting in her kitchen surrounded by her family's food and her mother's love, still feeling like she was losing her mind. I thought about Amy, two states away from anyone who could show up with a warm meal, figuring it out one granola bar at a time. And I thought about myself, reaching past the congee in the fridge for crackers because crackers required nothing of me.

Three women, three completely different support systems, and the same invisible gap between what our bodies needed and what we actually knew to give them.

What strikes me most, looking back, is not what we went through. It is what we did not know. None of us understood what was happening to our pelvic floors, our hormones, our nutrient stores, or our hydration. We were not careless or uninformed women. We just had not been told. And in the absence of the right information, we did what most new moms do: we got on with it and hoped for the best.

You now have the information we did not. And if you found any part of this book useful, there is a very good chance that someone in your life is either in this season right now or heading toward it. A friend who just had her baby. A colleague who is pregnant with her first. A sister who is further along than she expected to be in her recovery and cannot understand why.

Send this book their way. Whenever you have a spare moment, leaving a review on Amazon is one of the smallest things you can do with the biggest ripple. Another mom out there is searching for exactly this, and your words might be what helps her find it. That is the kind of thing Sofia, Amy, and I would have wanted someone to do for us.

Scan the QR code below to leave your review:

[QR CODE PLACEHOLDER]

Conclusion

There is a version of postpartum recovery that most of us were never shown. The one where someone sits down with you, explains what actually happened to your body during birth, and gives you practical, honest tools to help it heal. The one where you know why your pelvic floor feels the way it does, why you cannot think straight, why you are exhausted no matter how much you sleep, and why the crackers you have been surviving on are not enough. The one where nobody tells you to just rest and bounce back, because they understand that bouncing back is not how recovery works.

That version of postpartum recovery is what this book was built around.

We started with your body's most fundamental need after birth: reconnecting with your breath and your pelvic floor before anything else. Not to rush recovery, but to give it the right foundation. The movement hacks in Part I were designed to meet you exactly where you were, whether you were three weeks postpartum or three months, whether you had a vaginal birth or a C-section, whether you felt ready to move or were only just beginning to consider it. Every hack built on the one before it, and by the end of Part I, you had something most new moms never get: a genuine understanding of how your body works and what it needs to feel strong again.

Part II turned to the other half of recovery, the nourishment that makes movement sustainable and healing possible. We talked honestly about the difference between eating and actually nourishing yourself, about the nutrients your body is quietly running out of, about what the supplement industry is marketing to you and what actually deserves your money. We talked about food traditions from around the world, what they understood long before modern research caught up, and how real nourishment in the fourth trimester does not require a perfect kitchen, two free hands, or a full night of sleep to pull off.

You know more now. That is not a small thing. And if you want to go deeper on the emotional and mental side of this season, the hormonal shifts, the identity changes, the relationship dynamics, and the moments when new motherhood feels nothing like you expected, that is exactly what *The Essential Postpartum Care Toolkit* was written for. The two books were designed to work together, because recovering fully after birth means taking care of both your body and your mind.

If there is one thing I want you to carry forward from these thirteen hacks, it is permission. Permission to take your recovery seriously, to nourish yourself without guilt, to ask for help without apology, and to measure your progress in how you feel rather than how quickly you bounce back.

Some days you will feel like you are making real progress, and other days you will feel like you are back at the beginning. Both are part of the same process. Your body went through something extraordinary, and it deserves the same patience and care you give to everyone else in your life without question.

Be as gentle with yourself as you would be with any new mom you love. Show up for your own recovery the way you would show up for a friend who needed you. And on the days when it feels like too much, come back to the smallest hack you can manage, one breath, one nourishing meal, one glass of water, and let that be enough for today.

Thank you for trusting this book with your recovery. I wrote it for every mom who deserved better information and did not have it when she needed it most. I hope it found you at exactly the right time.

The hardest part was never the recovery. It was believing you deserved one. And from the other side of these pages, I am cheering for you louder than you know!

Glossary

Amaranth: An ancient grain with complete protein content and higher iron levels than most common grains. Used in postpartum recovery recipes for its nutrient density.

Amino acids: The building blocks of protein. Specific amino acids including glycine, proline, and lysine are essential for collagen production and tissue repair after birth.

Beta-glucan fiber: A type of soluble fiber found in oats, linked to stable blood sugar, sustained energy, and potential support for milk production in breastfeeding mothers.

Biotin: A B vitamin marketed heavily for postpartum hair loss. Hair loss after birth is caused by hormonal shifts rather than biotin deficiency in most cases.

Brewer's yeast: A nutritional supplement high in B vitamins, iron, and protein, commonly used as a galactagogue. Has a bitter taste that is best masked in smoothies or oatmeal.

C-section (Caesarean section): A surgical birth in which the baby is delivered through incisions in the abdomen and uterus. Recovery involves healing through seven layers of tissue and requires specific nutritional support.

Choline: An essential nutrient critical for brain function, liver health, and infant neurological development. Consistently underrepresented in both diet and post-natal supplements. Best dietary sources include eggs and organ meats.

Collagen: The most abundant structural protein in the body, forming the scaffold of skin, connective tissue, tendons, and healing wounds. Production requires adequate protein and vitamin C working together.

Cortisol: The body's primary stress hormone. Elevated by sleep deprivation, which is chronic postpartum. High cortisol disrupts electrolyte retention, mood regulation, and recovery.

DHA (Docosahexaenoic acid): An omega-3 fatty acid that forms approximately 30 percent of the brain's gray matter. Significantly depleted during pregnancy as the baby's brain development takes priority. Linked to postpartum mood, cognitive function, and breast milk quality.

Diastasis recti: The partial or complete separation of the rectus abdominis muscles along the midline of the abdomen. Common after pregnancy. Requires specific exercise modifications and should be assessed before progressing core training.

Diaphragm: The dome-shaped muscle beneath the lungs that drives breathing. Works in coordination with the pelvic floor and deep core muscles to stabilize the trunk. Central to the 360° Breath technique.

Electrolytes: Minerals including sodium, potassium, magnesium, calcium, and chloride that carry electrical charges in body fluids. Regulate hydration at the cellular level, nerve function, and muscle contractions. Depleted through breastfeeding, sweating, and postpartum night sweats.

Episiotomy: A surgical cut made in the perineum during vaginal delivery to facilitate birth. Requires tissue repair supported by adequate protein and vitamin C for proper healing.

EPA (Eicosapentaenoic acid): An omega-3 fatty acid with the most consistent antidepressant effects in postpartum studies. Found alongside DHA in fatty fish and fish oil supplements.

Ferritin: A protein that stores iron in the body. Serum ferritin levels are the most accurate measure of iron stores postpartum. Low ferritin is associated with fatigue, brain fog, and postpartum depression even before full anemia develops.

Fourth trimester: The first three months after birth, characterized by significant physical recovery, hormonal adjustment, and newborn care demands. A period of high nutritional need for the mother.

Galactagogue: Any food, herb, or supplement believed to support or increase breast milk production. Examples include oats, moringa, brewer's yeast, fenugreek, fennel, and sesame seeds. Evidence varies significantly between different galactagogues.

Gut-brain axis: The bidirectional communication network between the gastrointestinal tract and the brain, involving nerves, hormones, and immune signals. Approximately 95 percent of the body's serotonin is produced in the gut. Diet and gut microbiome health directly influence mood.

Hypothalamus: A region of the brain that regulates thirst, hunger, body temperature, hormone release, and mood. Triggers the thirst response alongside oxytocin release during breastfeeding.

Induction (labor induction): The use of medical interventions to start or stimulate labor before it begins naturally. Methods include medications and mechanical techniques.

Iodine: A mineral essential for thyroid hormone production, which regulates energy, metabolism, and mood. Breastfeeding significantly increases iodine requirements. One of the most commonly under-supplemented nutrients in postnatal formulas.

Iron: A mineral critical for oxygen transport in the blood. Significantly depleted during pregnancy and delivery. Iron deficiency postpartum is strongly associated with fatigue, brain fog, and postpartum depression.

Iron bisglycinate: A highly bioavailable and gentle form of supplemental iron where iron is bound to the amino acid glycine. Better absorbed and significantly easier on digestion than ferrous sulfate, making it the preferred form in postnatal supplements.

Kegel: A pelvic floor exercise involving repeated contraction and relaxation of the pelvic floor muscles. Named after Dr. Arnold Kegel. Kegels performed incorrectly or exclusively without relaxation can worsen symptoms rather than improve them.

Lactational amenorrhea: The temporary suppression of menstruation during breastfeeding. Reduces iron loss, which is why iron requirements are lower for breastfeeding women than during pregnancy.

Letdown reflex: The release of milk from the breast in response to the baby latching or other stimuli. Triggered by oxytocin. Accompanied by a surge in thirst in many breastfeeding mothers.

Magnesium: A mineral involved in over 300 enzymatic reactions including serotonin production, cortisol regulation, sleep quality, and nerve function. Commonly depleted during pregnancy. Deficiency is associated with increased anxiety, irritability, and postpartum depression risk.

Methylated folate (5-MTHF): The active, bioavailable form of folate that the body can use directly without conversion. Preferred over folic acid in postnatal supplements, particularly for women with the MTHFR gene variant who have difficulty converting folic acid.

Methylcobalamin: The most bioavailable and active form of vitamin B12. Preferred over cyanocobalamin in postnatal supplements as it is more readily used by the body without requiring conversion.

Matrescence: The psychological and identity transformation a woman undergoes when becoming a mother. A significant neurological and emotional process that accompanies the physical changes of the postpartum period.

Microbiome: The community of trillions of microorganisms living in and on the body, particularly the gut. Gut microbiome diversity influences mood, immune function, digestion, and nutrient absorption. Disrupted by birth, antibiotics, and hormonal changes.

Moringa: A plant whose leaves are used as a nutritional supplement and galactagogue. Has the strongest research backing of any food galactagogue, with studies showing it can increase breast milk volume by up to 400 milliliters per day.

Neuroplasticity: The brain's ability to reorganize and form new neural connections. Matrescence involves significant neuroplastic changes that support bonding, attunement, and caregiving.

Oxytocin: A hormone released during breastfeeding that triggers the letdown reflex and simultaneously activates thirst. Also plays a role in bonding, stress response, and uterine contractions during and after birth.

Pelvic floor: A hammock of muscles stretching from the pubic bone to the tailbone, supporting the bladder, uterus, and rectum. Significantly affected by pregnancy and birth regardless of delivery method.

Perineal tear: A tear in the tissue between the vaginal opening and the anus that can occur during vaginal delivery. Requires tissue repair supported by adequate protein and vitamin C.

Postnatal depletion: A state of physical, nutritional, and hormonal exhaustion that can persist months or years after birth if not adequately addressed. Characterized by fatigue, brain fog, mood instability, and nutrient deficiencies.

Postpartum anxiety (PPA): A mood disorder characterized by excessive worry, fear, and physical anxiety symptoms following birth. Linked to hormonal changes, sleep deprivation, and nutrient deficiencies including vitamin D, magnesium, and DHA.

Postpartum depression (PPD): A mood disorder involving persistent low mood, loss of interest, and difficulty functioning following birth. Affects approximately 10 to 20 percent of new mothers. Nutritional deficiencies can contribute to risk.

Prenatal vitamin: A multivitamin formulated to support pregnancy and fetal development. Often continued postpartum but may require adjustments as nutritional needs change after birth.

Prolactin: The hormone responsible for milk production. Released in response to nipple stimulation and suckling. Some galactagogues are believed to work by influencing prolactin levels.

Serotonin: A neurotransmitter involved in mood regulation, appetite, and sleep. Approximately 95 percent is produced in the gut. Production requires adequate tryptophan, B vitamins, and a healthy gut microbiome.

Synaptogenesis: The formation of new neural connections in the brain. Occurs significantly during the matrescence process and in the developing infant brain.

Telogen effluvium: The medical term for postpartum hair loss, caused by the sudden drop in estrogen after birth that shifts large numbers of hair follicles into a resting and shedding phase. Temporary and unrelated to biotin deficiency in most cases.

Third-party tested: A quality certification for supplements indicating that an independent organization has verified the product's contents, purity, and dosage accuracy. Look for NSF or USP certification when purchasing postnatal supplements.

360° Breath: A diaphragmatic breathing technique that expands the ribcage in all directions simultaneously, activating the deep core and pelvic floor. Forms the foundation of postpartum core reconnection in this book.

Vitamin D: A fat-soluble vitamin that functions as a neuroactive hormone. Found in fatty fish, egg yolks, and sunlight exposure. Deficiency is strongly associated with postpartum depression and is extremely common in new mothers who spend limited time outdoors.

Zuo yuezi: The traditional Chinese postpartum confinement practice lasting approximately one month after birth. Based on the principle of protecting the body's heat and energy during recovery. Includes specific warming foods, rest requirements, and movement restrictions.

ACKNOWLEDGEMENT

This book was born from the same personal season of exhaustion, learning, and quiet courage that shaped my first postpartum book, only this time, I went looking for the practical tools I wished someone had handed me for my body and what it needed to recover. It would never have made it into your hands without my people. To my husband and children, thank you for your patience, your hugs on the hard days, and your ability to bring laughter into even the messiest moments. You are the heart behind every word on these pages.

To my sister, my lifelong therapist in every sense of the word, thank you for holding space for me even while you are busy caring for your own clients. Your listening ear and steady support have been a lifeline more times than I can count. To my extended family, I am deeply grateful. I feel so lucky to have you to lean on when I needed help, encouragement, or simply a reminder that I am not alone.

I also want to speak directly to the moms who may not feel as supported. Some of you might be reading this in the quiet of the night, feeling worn out, scared, or wondering if this season will ever end. If that is you, I want this note of thanks to reach your heart too. You may feel alone, but you are not. I am always just an email away at info@kaceyquinnauthor.com, and it truly matters to me that you feel seen and heard.

Thank you, dear reader, for trusting me enough to walk beside you in your postpartum days. My hope is that these pages bring you comfort, practical help, and a little more kindness toward yourself. You deserve care just as much as the little one in your arms.

ALSO CREATED BY THE AUTHOR

The Essential Postpartum Toolkit Series

The Essential Postpartum Care Toolkit

El kit esencial de cuidado posparto

Anger Management for Parents

Anger Management for Parents Made Simple

Manejo de la ira para padres

The Our Family Project

A growing journal series designed to help families talk, listen, and grow together:

Our Family's Big Feelings Journal

Our Family's Adventure Journal

Our Family's Gratitude Journal

Our Family's Story Journal

Our Family's Bible Journal

Our Family: My Mom's Journal

Our Family: My Dad's Journal

All titles are available on Amazon. Scan QR code below to find the full catalog.

150

ABOUT THE AUTHOR

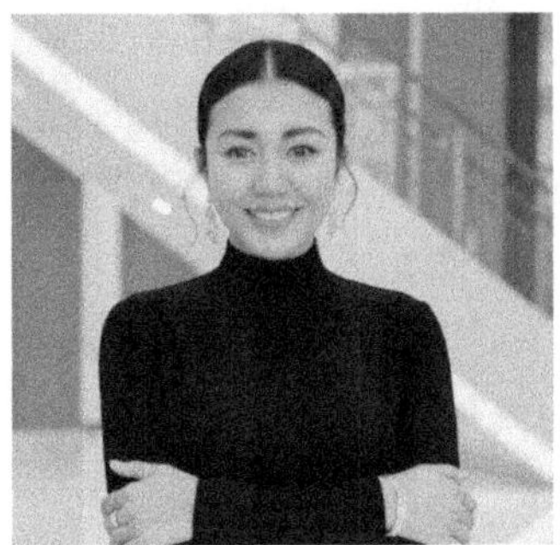

Kacey Quinn is a writer, mom, and gentle encourager of parents in the tender seasons of family life. She created "The Essential Postpartum Exercises and Nutrition Toolkit" to give new mothers the practical, honest tools they need to rebuild strength and nourish recovery in the weeks and months after birth, information she wishes she had found sooner herself.

Kacey believes that small, practical steps can create powerful change in a home. Through her books, she offers simple tools that fit into real family rhythms, not perfect ones. When she is not writing, you can find her laughing with her family, dreaming up new DIY projects, or curled up with a good book. She lives in the Atlanta area, where the kindness and sense of community continue to inspire her work with parents everywhere.

REFERENCES

Afshariani, Rahele, et al. 2019. "The Influence of Ergonomic Breastfeeding Training on Some Health Parameters in Infants and Mothers: A Randomized Controlled Trial." *Archives of Public Health* 77: 56. https://doi.org/10.1186/s13690-019-0373-x.

Aghajafari, Fariba, et al. 2018. "Association Between Maternal Serum 25-Hydroxyvitamin D Level and Pregnancy and Neonatal Outcomes." *BMC Pregnancy and Childbirth* 18 (1): 1–10. https://doi.org/10.1186/s12884-018-1702-2.

Beard, J. L., M. K. Hendricks, E. M. Perez, et al. 2005. "Maternal Iron Deficiency Anemia Affects Postpartum Emotions and Cognition." *Journal of Nutrition* 135 (2): 267–72. https://doi.org/10.1093/jn/135.2.267.

Bettinelli, Maria Enrica, et al. 2025. "Moringa oleifera Supplementation as a Natural Galactagogue: A Systematic Review on Its Role in Supporting Milk Volume and Prolactin Levels." *Nutrients* 17 (12): 1989. https://doi.org/10.3390/nu17121989.

Carr, Anitra C., and Silvia Maggini. 2017. "Vitamin C and Immune Function." *Nutrients* 9 (11): 1211. https://doi.org/10.3390/nu9111211.

Dowling, Donna A., et al. 2023. "Breastfeeding Posture and Musculoskeletal Pain in Lactating Mothers." *Breastfeeding Medicine* 17: 926–31. https://doi.org/10.1089/bfm.2022.0138.

Ellsworth-Bowers, E. R., and E. J. Corwin. 2012. "Nutrition and the Psychoneuroimmunology of Postpartum Depression." *Nutrition Research Reviews* 25 (1): 180–92. https://doi.org/10.1017/S0954422412000091.

Grand View Research. 2024. "Postpartum Health Supplements Market Size, Share and Trends Analysis Report." https://www.grandviewresearch.com/industry-analysis/postpartum-health-supplements-market-report.

Hansraj, Kenneth K. 2014. "Assessment of Stresses in the Cervical Spine Caused by Posture and Position of the Head." *Surgical Technology International* 25: 277–79. https://pubmed.ncbi.nlm.nih.gov/25393825/.

Hoekzema, Elseline, et al. 2017. "Pregnancy Leads to Long-Lasting Changes in Human Brain Structure." *Nature Neuroscience* 20 (2): 287–96. https://doi.org/10.1038/nn.4458.

Hsu, Mei-Chi, Ching-Yun Tung, and Hsi-En Chen. 2018. "Omega-3 Polyunsaturated Fatty Acid Supplementation in Prevention and Treatment of Maternal Depression: Putative Mechanism and Recommendation." *Journal of Affective Disorders* 238: 47–61. https://doi.org/10.1016/j.jad.2018.05.018.

Innis, Sheila M. 2003. "Perinatal Biochemistry and Physiology of Long-Chain Polyunsaturated Fatty Acids." *Journal of Pediatrics* 143 (4 Suppl): S1–8. https://doi.org/10.1067/s0022-3476(03)00396-2.

Keats, Emily C., et al. 2025. "Dietary Supplements in Pregnancy and Postpartum: Evidence, Safety Challenges and a Precision Nutrition Framework." *Antioxidants* 15 (1): 57. https://doi.org/10.3390/antiox15010057.

Levant, Beth. 2011. "N-3 (Omega-3) Fatty Acids in Postpartum Depression: Implications for Prevention and Treatment." *Depression Research and Treatment* 2011: 467349. https://doi.org/10.1155/2011/467349.

Marshall, Natalie E., Barbara Abrams, Linda A. Barbour, et al. 2022. "The Importance of Nutrition in Pregnancy and Lactation: Lifelong Consequences." *American Journal of Obstetrics and Gynecology* 226 (5): 607–32. https://doi.org/10.1016/j.ajog.2021.12.035.

Matsunaga, Michiko, et al. 2025. "Gut Microbiota and Diet as Contributing Factors to Postpartum Depression in Japanese Mothers." *PNAS Nexus* 4 (1). https://doi.org/10.1093/pnasnexus/pgae566.

McGill, Stuart. 2015. *Back Mechanic: The Secrets to a Healthy Spine Your Doctor Isn't Telling You.* Backfitpro Inc.

Michaud, F., et al. 2021. "Lower Back Injury Prevention and Sensitization of Hip Hinge with Neutral Spine Using Wearable Sensors during Lifting Exercises." *Sensors* 21 (16): 5487. https://doi.org/10.3390/s21165487.

Murray-Kolb, Laura E., and John L. Beard. 2007. "Iron Treatment Normalizes Cognitive Functioning in Young Women." *American Journal of Clinical Nutrition* 85 (3): 778–87. https://doi.org/10.1093/ajcn/85.3.778.

Pentland, Veronica, et al. 2021. "Does Walking Reduce Postpartum Depressive Symptoms? A Systematic Review and Meta-Analysis of Randomized Controlled Trials." *Journal of Women's Health* 30 (12): 1666–75. https://doi.org/10.1089/jwh.2021.0296.

Pullar, Juliet M., Anitra C. Carr, and Margreet C. M. Vissers. 2017. "The Roles of Vitamin C in Skin Health." *Nutrients* 9 (8): 866. https://doi.org/10.3390/nu9080866.

Ramsey, Drew. 2021. *Eat to Beat Depression and Anxiety.* New York: HarperWave.

Reiman, M. P., et al. 2012. "Gluteal Muscle Activation During Common Therapeutic Exercises." *Journal of Orthopaedic and Sports Physical Therapy* 39 (7): 532–40. https://doi.org/10.2519/jospt.2009.2796.

Ryan, Rachel A., et al. 2023. "Use of Galactagogues to Increase Milk Production Among Breastfeeding Mothers in the United States: A Descriptive Study." *Journal of the Academy of Nutrition and Dietetics* 123 (8): 1144–53. https://doi.org/10.1016/j.jand.2023.05.010.

Sahrmann, Shirley A. 2023. "Exercise Won't Change the Way You Move." Interview by Tim Ferriss. *The Tim Ferriss Show*, Episode 685. August 7, 2023. https://tim.blog/2023/08/04/dr-shirley-sahrmann/.

Sebastiani, Giorgia, et al. 2024. "Nutritional Status of Breastfeeding Mothers and Impact of Diet and Dietary Supplementation on Human Milk Composition: A Narrative Review." *Nutrients* 16 (2): 285. https://doi.org/10.3390/nu16020285.

Semba, Richard D., and Susan E. Juul. 1997. "Electrolyte Composition of Human Breast Milk Beyond the Early Postpartum Period." *Acta Paediatrica* 86 (9): 1007–8. https://doi.org/10.1111/j.1651-2227.1997.tb15187.x.

Shoulders, Matthew D., and Ronald T. Raines. 2009. "Collagen Structure and Stability." *Annual Review of Biochemistry* 78: 929–58. https://doi.org/10.1146/annurev.biochem.77.032207.120833.

Smith, Heather. 2023. "Postpartum Exercise: Getting Started After Giving Birth." Hinge Health. https://www.hingehealth.com/resources/articles/postpartum-exercise-getting-started/.

Stone, Jennifer. 2021. "Physical Therapy in Addition to Standard of Care Improves Patient Satisfaction and Recovery Post-Cesarean Section." *Journal of Women's Health Physical Therapy*. MU Health Care, Mizzou Therapy Services. https://www.muhealth.org/our-stories/physical-therapy-after-c-section-improves-outcomes.

Tziatzios, Georgios, et al. 2024. "Investigating Water Balance as a Nutritional Determinant in Breastfeeding: A Comparative Study of Water Consumption Patterns and Influencing Factors." *Nutrients* 16 (13): 2056. https://doi.org/10.3390/nu16132056.

van Reijn-Baggen, Daniëlle A., Ingrid J. M. Han-Geurts, Petra J. Voorham-van der Zalm, Rob C. M. Pelger, Caroline H. A. C. Hagenaars-van Miert, and Ellen T. M. Laan. 2022. "Pelvic Floor Physical Therapy for Pelvic Floor Hypertonicity: A Systematic Review of Treatment Efficacy." *Sexual Medicine Reviews* 10 (2): 209–30. https://doi.org/10.1016/j.sxmr.2021.03.002.

Wiebe, Julie. 2013. "Progressive Exercises for Post-Pregnancy." *NASM Blog*. National Academy of Sports Medicine. https://blog.nasm.org/progressive-exercises-for-post-pregnancy.

Yuan, Ye, et al. 2024. "The Association Between Vitamin D Deficiency and Perinatal Depression: A Systematic Review and Meta-Analysis." *Alpha Psychiatry* 25 (6): 669–675. https://doi.org/10.5152/alphapsychiatry.2024.241527.

Zeisel, Steven H. 2006. "Choline: Critical Role During Fetal Development and Dietary Requirements in Adults." *Annual Review of Nutrition* 26: 229–50. https://doi.org/10.1146/annurev.nutr.26.061505.111156.

* 9 7 8 1 9 6 8 3 5 4 2 6 8 *